MW01485118

Is There
A Doctor In The House?

Common Sense Medical Insights And Anecdotes
From A Veteran Family Physician

By Dr. Glenn M. Cosh

Copyright 2013 by Dr. Glenn M. Cosh

All Rights Reserved

No part of this book may be reproduced in any form without prior permission from the author, except by a reviewer who may quote brief passages in review.

Zest Publishing

Second Edition

Library of Congress Catalogue Card Number TX 7-815-428

ISBN 978-0-578-11884-0
Printed in the USA

Other books by Dr. Glenn M. Cosh
A New Customized Prescription for Cycling
Cycling in the Slow Lane

Cover design and manuscript layout by
Stony Ridge Studios

This book is dedicated to the hundreds of thousands of physicians, of all degrees and specialties, who adhere to the unconditional commitment to reinforce the importance and significance of our patient's lives.

Thanks to my colleagues, friends and wife Erin for encouraging me to pursue this book. Also a special recognition to my son Greg, a Hollywood film writer and director, for his help and support with the manuscript.

CONTENTS

Foreword

My wife and I, along with another couple, were in attendance at a play at the historic Central City Opera House, Colorado. The leading actor was none other than Don Ameche, famous Hollywood actor and movie star. During the first act, there was a cry from the audience that a man was having a heart attack. The play stopped, and Mr. Ameche asked, "Is there a doctor in the house?" Our friends quickly pointed to me, whereupon Mr. Ameche said thanks, and continued with the performance. However, the play was over for me; after attending to the heart patient, I ended up assisting several other patrons that also fell ill that warm evening. Incidentally, although I only saw one act that evening, hearing Don Ameche ask, "Is there a doctor in the house?" more than made up for it. It certainly wasn't the first, or last time, I would hear that question.

A physician's education is based on evidence-based medicine. It is rooted in the judicious use of the best information available, while making decisions about the care of an individual patient. It integrates clinical expertise, the best available research, and the values of a patient. Nevertheless, at times, this education can distract the physician from thinking outside the box, along with using a little common sense, which can potentially result in a substantial reduction in health care cost. For example, let's say a young male complaining of a recent rapid pulse, palpitations and nervousness is seen in the emergency room. He denies taking drugs. By the book he might get an electrocardiogram and blood workup, all of which come back as normal. He is discharged and told to follow up with a physician. Depending on the hospital, his total emergency room bill could total $3,813.67: Metabolic panel $329.67, Assay of magnesium $246.97, CBC $219.66, Chest X-ray $464.08, Place needle in vein $129.35, ER visit $1,457.04, Electrocardiogram $383.90, and ER doctor $583.00. The following week he sees a family physician that his boss recommended. By taking a thorough history and with some common sense, the physician inquires about recent events occurring in his life. It's found he's started working for a fast food chain. Further questioning reveals he's entitled to free food and drinks. He admits to drinking more than a dozen caffeinated drinks a day. Simply by factoring in his age, profession, and recent diet change, he's advised to gradually wean himself off caffeine over the next 3-4 weeks. A follow up call two weeks later revealed his rapid pulse and nervousness had subsided. Total cost: less than $100.

Another example involved a stocky middle-aged male who recently had been treated by another health care provider. He'd been complaining of recent lower back pain that radiated down his left leg. He denied any recent lifting or injury to his back. With no improvement after seven office visits, and spending over $800, including x-rays, he decided to see a family physician on the recommendation of a friend. With a detailed history, the physician found that as a regional sales representative, the patient was driving up to four hours a day. He'd also recently purchased a new Mercedes with tight-fitting bucket seats. Using a little common sense the physician also noticed a large wallet in his left back pocket. By simply having the patient remove his wallet while driving, the back symptoms quickly subsided. Total cost: less than $100.

When dealing with their personal health, patients also need to use common sense. In physics, Sir. Isaac Newton's 3rd law of motion states for every action, there is an equal and opposite reaction. In everyday life, we experience this law. I won't go to work today. The counter reaction being, I may loose my job. The same type of comparison can also apply to medicine. I won't take my insulin. The counter reaction is, I not only risk my health, but also my life. Common sense therefore dictates that it's in my best interest to take my insulin. Any other course of action on my part would be counterproductive, and possibly fatal.

Sometimes we make medicine way too complicated. Case in point: an elderly female student complains she's seeing spots. The practitioner proceeds with a full eye exam, all of which is normal. Had the practitioner quizzed her on recent activities, she would have told him she had just spray painted some of her pottery. By examining her glasses first, he would have graciously cleaned them and returned her clear vision, minus the exam.

Prior to a definitive diagnosis, health professionals can increase a patient's stress and anxiety by giving them the worst-case scenario. A professional bull rider sees a urologist with a painful testicle. Following the exam, the doctor curtly informs the patient that it's probably cancer, and he may die from it. The bull rider has a syncope reaction and lands on the doctor's floor— not from the big bad bull, but from an insensitive doctor.

If you listen to a patient long enough, the chances are they will give you the diagnoses. A man in this 30's shows up at the emergency room with vague chest discomfort. With scant medical history, the staff gets an EKG, chest X-ray, blood panel, all of which are normal. The patient is referred to his family physician for follow-up, without a diagnosis. His family doctor sees him the following day, inquiring in detail what had preceded the days prior to the chest discomfort. Nothing, except that he and his wife went shopping at the local mall. The patient recalls getting a cholesterol test for $10, was told his cholesterol was 250, and that probably put him at risk for a heart attack. His dinner that evening was sausage and sauerkraut. Incomplete blood test + invalid suggestion + anxiety + gaseous meal + indigestion and chest discomfort + ER visit + inadequate history = big bill with no diagnoses.

Sometimes common sense is lacking even in the ivory towers of medical research. While attending a medical meeting years ago, the speaker announced that a new hypertensive drug (beta blocker), after two years of use, improved the survival rate of patients with heart disease significantly, but didn't recommend it beyond the two years, even though no adverse side effects were noted. After asking him why not continue with the drug beyond that period, his response was that it needed more time for investigation. With that logic, you're potentially denying every heart patient the advantage of a better survival outcome because of a technical research requirement.

Back in the 60's, a pharmaceutical company representative detailed me on a new IUD (intra uterine device utilized for birth control). On examination, common sense told me this device could have potential harmful effects to the patient, because of its design, so I choose not use it on my female patients. The next thing I knew, several gynecologists from the medical school called to inform me I was premature in not using it. I told them to call me back after it was on the market awhile; I didn't trust their judgment. Without mentioning the product, it was taken off the market years later. It had caused multiple deaths, and the company was sued. By the way, I was never called back from those gynecologists and the pharmaceutical representative never returned to my office.

That same common sense utilized in patient-physician interactions is also applicable to how medical care has evolved over the last half century. It can also be applied to lowering medical costs, choosing the right physician, understanding our bodies, and how to respond to our everyday common medical, physical, emotional, and spiritual problems.

Is There A Doctor In The House?

CHAPTER 1

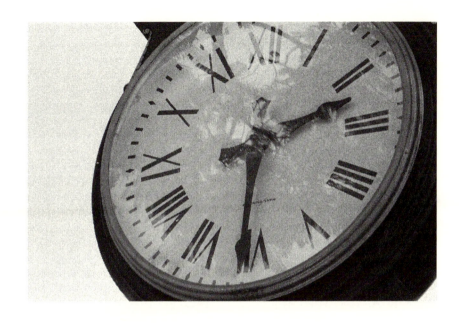

CHARLES DICKENS MEDICINE
MEDICAL CARE IN THE USA:
PAST, PRESENT, AND FUTURE TENSE

Charles Dickens may have been looking into the future of medicine in the United States when he said, "A person who can't pay gets another person who can't pay to guarantee that he can pay. Like a person with two wooden legs getting another person with two wooden legs to guarantee that he has got two natural legs, it won't make either of them able to do a walking match."

PAST TENSE

Past tense medical care (circa 19th century thru 1965) was a simpler time, when patients were seen by their personal physician, usually a GP (General Practitioner) and paid their bill by cash or check. For those with insurance (Blue Cross/ Blue shield for the most part), the doctor would bill the insurance company. The GP would correlate, or quarterback, their entire patient needs; including office visits, house calls, and hospital visits. If specialists were needed, he would still oversee the patients total care. Physician's overhead was approximately 30%, and office visit charges were minimal. For patients who were out of work or behind with their bills, most physicians would accept less, or the doctor would simply write off the bill. Many physicians would also volunteer at medical indigent clinics, serving the homeless and transients. Various religious groups supported these clinics. Additional support came from hospitals, medical societies, and pharmaceutical companies, supplying free samples to those patients.

PRESENT TENSE

Today, we are in an environment in which too many things have an impact on what physicians can and cannot do. Physicians lose both autonomy and control as they move from ownership of their own practices to being employees of groups or hospitals. Also, the majority of primary care physicians were now known as FP (Family Physicians), a designation that requires several additional years of training and certification.

Also we saw the introduction of hospitalist (hospital based physicians) now caring for hospitalized patients, especially in urban hospitals. A potential problem arises when the discharged patient is given prescriptions and instructions from the treating hospital physician, prior to informing the primary care physician. Case in point: the family physician referred a patient with pulmonary emboli to the hospital. After appropriate care, the hospitalists and pulmonologist discharged the patient. Failing to confer with each other, both gave the patient the same blood thinning prescription. A week later the patient was again hospitalized with internal bleeding.

Medical care, as we knew it, no longer exists, it has become politically and financially motivated in recent times. Physicians are frequently caught between the pathway to serve the needy, but also belonging to powerful vested interest corporations, which by their structure are sensitive to bottom line profits. Across the nation there exist a cadre of concerned family physicians who quietly, compassionately, and altruistically initiate efforts to aid the medically indigent—those who have fallen through the cracks in the American dream. Perhaps as physicians, we can garner a better perspective of our destiny by reviewing the biblical parable about the traveler who was beaten and robbed on his journey from Jerusalem to Jericho. The Priest who denied he existed, and the Levite who wanted to legislate the job to others, bypassed him. However, it was the Good Samaritan who assisted the wounded traveler.

Beginning for the most part in the late 60's, physicians were enticed to join third party insurance companies. They came to be known as Health

Maintenance Organizations (HMO's) and Independent Practice Associations (IPA's). The HMOs would sign a capitation contract with the physicians, who would then be paid a flat fee for each patient. The IPA's were merely a group of physicians that would contract with an HMO. These insurance companies would then contract with different employer groups. At the discretion of their employer, the patient would subscribe to a group's insurance medical plan. There was a small co-pay charge the patient had to pay to their doctor for each visit. There were downsides for both the physician and the patient. The doctor had to belong to that particular insurance plan, thereby accepting a discounted fee, and was forced to refer the patient to the hospital and specialist designated by the insurance carrier. Patients were forced to either find another doctor, or pressure their long time regular doctor to join with their insurance group.

With the insurance groups now taking a third of every health care dollar, (thus increasing the cost of health care), and for those patients without group insurance, the number of uninsured and medically indigent quickly rose to a third of our population. As a result, we saw an increase in the Medicaid population.

Physicians were now under additional government and insurance intervention and red tape. This included more paperwork, spending more time in front of a computer, and ultimately, less time with a patient. With office overhead reaching 60%, they felt more inclined to treat medicine as a business rather than a compassionate service to their patients.

The argument can also be made that increased malpractice rates, coupled with too many unnecessary high cost procedures, were perhaps raising medical costs in the US to over $7000 per person—which is unsustainable. The list goes on. The question is, how did we allow this to spiral out of control? Perhaps it was a gradual accumulation of honest and dishonest misjudgments over time. It's a bit like putting a frog in tepid water, and gradually increasing the temperature. Before it knows what's happened, the poor frog will eventually die as the temperature slowly reaches the boiling point.

Greed has played perhaps the biggest role in this fiasco. Corporate mentally, along with the bean counters, drove medical care into the moneychanger's arena, with many an insurance CEO becoming a multimillionaire.

The downside of new medical technology (MRI and CAT scans to name but a few) is the excessive cost of the equipment. Paying for this hi-tech equipment tempted many hospitals and doctors to over-prescribe their use. There's also a wide disparity between what hospitals charge for the same procedure. Recently, The Associated Press showed the cost for an appendectomy ranged between $1,500 to $180,000. Our health care dollars can't sustain such massive disparities.

Because there's big money in the healthcare marketplace, there's fierce competition between hospitals for their share of the pie. Hospitals are staking out territory in each other's backyard. It's like a game of checkers, where they leapfrog over each other's turf to see who can claim the most prestige and the biggest piece of the healthcare dollar. Back in the 70's, two hospitals that I was on staff with were just a few miles apart. Initially, they joined forces and combined both staffs into one. Additional cooperation included not duplicating expensive equipment, and utilizing one hospital for obstetrics, while the other would focus on neurosurgery. For years this honeymoon worked out well, saving money that benefited both doctors and patients. However, philosophical differences, prestige, and perhaps competing for the medical dollar ended that cooperation. Because both were nonprofits, they plowed their revenues into massive expansions and hiring doctors. Problems arise when the hospital employs the doctors and also has a pact with the insurance company, and patient protection is compromised.

Adding to the stew were government regulations from HIPAA (Health Insurance Portability Accountability Act)—patient privacy rule. This over-regulating government agency, lacking common sense, earned the nickname "HYPER" by many physicians. A patient of mine, whom we will call "Bob", offers an example of HIPAA's lack of common sense. A neighbor found Bob's elderly father unconscious, and had him taken to a local hospital in New Jersey. Bob called the hospital, notifying them of his father's medications, and inquiring about his condition. He was informed that HIPAA would not allow the hospital to give that information out, unless he had his unconscious father's permission!

The argument for EMR (mandatory electronic medical records) is logical and has merit. It's supposed to reduce cost, errors, redundant tests, dangerous drug interactions, and illegible handwriting. But several studies have shown that EMRs have not improved patient outcomes, nor saved money. The technology has become a faceless piece of equipment contradicting the decisions a physician might make. Furthermore, the EMR can increase insurance company denials of a treatment plan a physician may want. For example, a dermatologist needs to surgically (Mohs procedure) remove two biopsied basal cell cancerous legions from an elderly patient with heart disease that resides in a rural area 60 miles from the office. The EMR however, only approved one surgical procedure per visit, thus requiring the patient to make an additional stressful trip for the second surgery.

Essentially, the physician's personal commitment to a patient, along with their common sense judgment based on real life experience with that patient, is overridden by the EMR. There are also potential problems with the EMR vendors and EMR templates that do not match exactly what that particular patient is being treated for.

With the introduction of newly funded federal health programs, the traditional doctor-patient relationship now has two additional dictatorial partners—insurance companies and state/federal governments. The combined total cost for these programs exceeded 2.7 trillion dollars in 2010, according to the Associated Press.

When factoring in the cost of medical care, defining quality care, rationing it, and then deciding who ultimately shoulders the responsibility for dispensing it, you create a witch's brew. Bottom line—we will have too many cooks stirring the cauldron, so to speak. The unfortunate part is that it will take a lot longer to fix it than it took to break it.

Aside from overbearing bureaucracy, greed has also infiltrated medicine. Lawyers flood the airways persuading patients to join in class action lawsuits against just about every drug on the market. Pharmaceutical companies are now focusing their marketing not so much on physicians, but on TV and magazines, advertising directly to the patients—"hey shouldn't everyone be on ED (erectile dysfunction) meds?" You might be outside the norm, if you don't.

We can also add some celebrity TV physicians to the money market. Unquestionably, the majority of these programs provide useful information to their viewers; however, many more have been trivialized into hocking everything from skin creams to tea leaves from Spain.

We can't, nor should we set our clocks back, but we can insist on a more common sense approach to healthcare. Let's collectively put greed and politics in last place, not first, when addressing our health care needs. We need less cooks, and crooks, in the kitchen.

One feasible idea put forth has been to create an ethics committee composed of grassroots primary care physicians, common sense economists, and non-partisan patient representatives (all with a history of volunteering and leadership experience), that would advise both government and insurance agencies how best to assist the healthcare industry—somewhat similar to the Bowles-Simpson Plan (a select bipartisan panel of US congressional leaders to assist our country with it's debt crises). Could it work? Definitely, but will it garner the same resistance that the Bowles-Simpson Plan ran into? Probably, because the government and corporate insurance companies want total control of the health care industry, rather than take some common sense advice from the providers, even if it means being deliberately deceptive to achieve that goal.

FUTURE TENSE

Future tense medicine is perhaps both frightening and hopeful, or as Dickens might say in retrospect, "It was the best of times, it was the worst of times." The good news is the ever-evolving technology that's being pioneered in medicine. Everything from genome and stem cell science to newer vaccines and cancer-fighting drugs are but a few examples to look forward to. There will be greater advances in preventive care, with improved school lunch programs and greater emphases on daily physical activities. The frightening part is that we need to initiate drastic changes now in our children's diets and their lack of physical activity. If no action is taken, we can look forward to one in three Americans being diabetic by 2050. The CDC (Centers for Disease Control) states that by exercising daily, and using proper diet, diabetes can be reduced by 58%.

Dickens was quoted as saying "There is a wisdom of the head, and a wisdom of the heart." If we look to the past, using a little common sense, we might anticipate the future with a transcendental sense and create a new model of delivering medical care with compassion, not driven by bean counters or bottom line profits, especially at the corporate level. A new maze of flowcharts to better assist the patients, coupled with an integrated care approach that is timely and efficient, would be a step in the right direction. For a model to be sustainable, it needs to be transparent, with a moral compass. This will require a fair reimbursement plan derived from the bottom up, not passed down by the government or corporate insurance companies. Finally, our current hi-tech - hi-cost 21st Century medical care could use an infusion of low-tech - low-cost common sense medicine. This includes a common sense patient/doctor relationship, where time for a thorough history and physical examination is allowed. Robotic medicine will never replace this essential part of medicine, or as Dickens himself put it, "Electric communication will never be a substitute for the face of someone who with their soul encourages another person to be brave and true."

CHAPTER 2

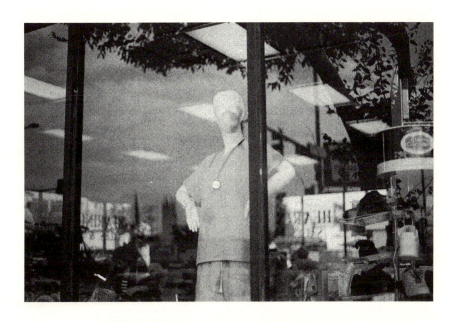

COMMON SENSE GUIDELINES
FOR CHOOSING A PHYSICIAN

Like many other professions, physicians are in the business of providing a service. They are given higher standards to adhere to than perhaps other service providers, because their decisions affect human lives. They rely on a support team of receptionists, nurses, technicians, specialists and therapists. Their training and experience place them in a unique position to predict their patient's future health needs, based on the patients past history, and present health status, somewhat analogous to Charles Dickens' stories of past, present, and future tense. For example, a physician sees a 48 year-old male with advanced emphysema (chronic lung disorder, resulting in breathing impairment) and a history of smoking two packs of cigarettes a day in treatment room 1, then sees a 21 year-old male with a history of smoking two packs of cigarettes a day in treatment room 2. It's reasonable for the physician to predict that he'll see the 21 year-old in 27 years or less in a similar condition as the 48 year-old patient in room 1, if no lifestyle changes are made. As physicians, we have the opportunity in the present to motivate the 21 year-old to avoid the past mistakes of the 48 year old, and help shape a brighter future in the process.

As with all professions, there are the good, the bad and the ugly. No one degree (D.O./M.D), or specialty, is immune from bad docs. Criteria for a good doc include competency, staying current, having sound ethics, being available to listen, being compassionate, being empathic, and if in doubt, willing to ask for consultation. I'm proud to say that in my four plus decades of practice, I've found that the overwhelming majority of physicians are good. They've experienced the joy of bringing a new life into this world, and holding the hands of those departing. They've shared a family's hardships, as well as their blessings in life, and been humbled beyond words by patients expressing their gratitude for the care they've given, and being called their friend. The bad doc usually lacks several of the above attributes.

There are docs who occasionally succumb to the "white-lie scenario" or gray area—"Hey; I'm not doing anything illegally or grossly wrong." Case in point: one of my patient's mothers was visiting from Miami, and was seen by me for a minor medical problem. After the exam, I gave her the discharge form and instructed her to check out at the front office. She then handed me a $20 dollar bill, which I said no to; the front office will handle it. She then informed me that her doc back home always accepted a tip. Although it's completely acceptable at your local restaurant, I find it unethical in medicine. We are placed in a position of responsibility for our patients, and should never be temped to take advantage of their generosity. When I first went into practice in the mid-60s, one of my elderly widowed patients asked if she could add me to her will, because she had no other family to give her assets to. In declining the offer, I suggested she talk it over with her accountant and find a suitable charity to give it to. I thought it a bit strange, and couldn't believe a physician would ever accept such an offer, until years later when another one of my patients told me her wealthy widowed aunt gave her multi million-dollar estate to her personal physician.

The ugly docs are the ones we usually see exposed in the media falsifying visits and charges, practicing with extreme medical incompetence, operating on a wrong part of the body, or prescribing narcotics for profit, like those signing off on the medical marijuana scams. Some have succumbed to the influence of money from their celebrity patients (Elvis Presley and Michael Jackson), resulting in tragedy.

In addition to using common sense when dealing with your medical problems, one needs to apply the same common sense when selecting a good physician.

Prior to selecting a doc, call the local medical society, medical board or scan the Internet for recommendations. Beware of physicians using excessive advertising. Those costs are usually made up for with high-cost and high-volume practices. Certainly personal references are the strongest and most reliable source for finding a good doc. However, third party medicine today may negate all the above. If your insurance only allows you to see a doc you haven't researched or know, then you may be on shaky ground until you feel comfortable with that particular doc.

Generally your first visit to the office is your first clue to acquiring a level of comfort with the physician. If you get a curt or unfriendly response from the front desk, it may suggest the office staff and doc won't be any better. That added stress only increases your fear that your problem is more serious than you anticipated. This is particularly true if you cannot be seen for several weeks, or not even given the option to talk to a nurse. In a panic, you might refer yourself to an emergency room, where you could be subject to unnecessary cost and testing.

Ideally on your first visit, it's only you and the physician in the room. Getting your medical history requires adequate time, which in time leads to a more accurate diagnosis. Beware of the doc who doesn't have time to take an adequate history. The legendary physician, Dr. Charles Mayo, always instructed his medical students on the importance of taking a proper history. He was often quoted as saying, "If you allow the patient enough time to talk, they will tell you the diagnosis". A doc, who has the patience to sit and smile while taking the history, will usually get a more accurate diagnosis for the patient. An incomplete history may lead the doc to prematurely order unnecessary tests. Case in point: a radiologist colleague told me he occasionally receives an order to perform a CAT scan for appendicitis, only to learn the patient previously had an appendectomy. Due to an incomplete history, the doc creates a flagrant mistake and unnecessary cost. A good doc will listen to all of the patient's concerns, and systematically place them in order of immediate priority, rescheduling the least serious for a future visit. Avoid the doc who watches the clock, and is anxious to leave the room before you've had all your concerns addressed. Many a time, I've had patients say as they're leaving the treatment room, "Hey doc, by the way, I've noticed I have trouble breathing while climbing stairs lately", almost as an afterthought—similar to Peter Falk in *Columbo* saying "By the way sir, I have one more question for you." Those patients are brought back to the treatment room for further evaluation.

Along with a thorough history, a complete physical examination and evaluation of any test results should be initiated before an actual diagnosis can be made. This of course means additional time may be required to have the medical problem solved. Factors influencing incorrect diagnosis include an inadequate physical and history, a lab error, or a communication problem amongst the medical team. This is not only a travesty for the patient, but adds measurably to the cost of medical care. Your physician needs to be qualified to connect all the dots to ensure the best possible diagnosis and treatment for you as a patient.

Finally, don't hesitate to ask questions or challenge your doctor if you're not comfortable with their diagnosis or treatment. If your health issue is too complex, or you're confused with a diagnosis or treatment plan, don't hesitate to get another opinion.

CHAPTER 3

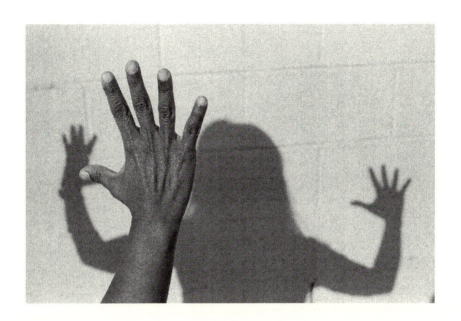

UNDERSTANDING OUR BODIES

A number of years ago I was invited to teach fifth graders basic human physiology. The approach I took was to relate how our bodily functions compared to that of their family car. It turned out to be a very lively, stimulating, humorous and fun experience for both the students and myself.

In keeping with this same theme, I'll assess our basic human systems in a similar way with our mechanical world. Utilizing some common sense, I'll keep the focus on the most common medical events that affect most of our lives. This will include our pipes (vascular), pump (heart), framework (muscular-skeleton system), computer (brain and nerves), rust (cancer), fuel (digestive and lungs), and reproduction (sex). I'll share the incidents I've experience in over four decades of practicing family medicine as they relate to our physiology. I'll attempt to avoid all the technical jargon that can already be found in the countless other publications on the subject. Keep in mind, this is not designed to be a paradigm for all patients or subject matter; each individual should rely on their personal physician for final judgment relating to their health needs.

"I-BRAIN"

A COMMON SENSE APPROACH TO OUR COMPUTER
(BRAIN and NERVES)

If you are impressed with your I-Pad, I-Phone, I-Mac, I-Pod or any other electronic device, you will be blown away by how much more the human brain can do. If the capacity of your computer is the size of a marble, then your brain's capacity is the size of a basketball. It's also responsive to all of our five senses—sight, smell, taste, hearing, and touch. You can place your computer on sleep phase, but it doesn't dream like your brain, which stays active 24-7, both in the conscious and sub-conscious state. Our brain determines who we are as people—our intellect, character, personality, values, ambitions, morality, and much more. Our nerves are merely the venue to keep

30

our bodies and brain connected. Our body is constantly talking to the brain, and our brain is constantly talking back to the body. A gastroenterologist colleague told me about one of his associates that had some abdominal pain and was convinced it was cancer. After being told his exam was completely normal, the pain was instantly gone. In other words, the subconscious part of his brain needed that reassurance to cancel the phantom pain he was experiencing.

Though we pride ourselves in our ability to multitask, we usually are focused on one item at a time, while subconsciously keeping our "back burners" in overload. That's why one moment you're enjoying a pleasant ride in the countryside and the next you're enraged, because you were just cut off by another driver. When we're upset, the last incidence you were focused on is reshuffled to your "back burner". Prior to 8:46 AM (EST) on September 11th 2001 or 9/11, the country was focused on their daily routines. Shortly thereafter, we witnessed the American Airlines passenger jet crashing into the North Tower of the World Trade Center, on our TVs. Suddenly, our focus on our daily routines was out the window. That's why, when you're over focused on something that's upsetting you, its beneficial to quickly redirect your focus into something that is pleasant...be it listening to music, taking a walk, or watching your favorite show on TV. For one overworked mother of eight, it was focusing on crossword puzzles.

Somewhat akin to your computer breaking down, our brain and nerves can also misfire, or get a virus. They also require maintenance and treatment. As with the rest of our body, good care requires some daily discipline and common sense—proper diet, rest, adequate hours of sleep, fun, contentment, and being at peace with yourself. How do you find that peace? Stop and analyze every aspect of yourself. Start with your physical body. Do you accept yourself in your present state, or are you attempting to mirror your image to someone else's? Early in my practice, I saw an attractive professional model for a small facial blemish that I had difficulty seeing. I reassured her no pathology was present, and that it wasn't distracting to her appearance, but her perception was that it made her unattractive. Instead of being pleased with her natural beauty, she saw herself as an ugly duckling.

Do you accept that you're intellectually competent, and stay informed, or do you feel inferior, and not care? Frequently, I see very intelligent and informed patients, who never advanced their education for any number of reasons, carry the perception that they are dumb. One bright, middle-aged female patient thought she was too old to further her education. She was frustrated with her incompetent boss and her lack of advancement at work. I encouraged her to take night classes at the local community college. Six years later, she had her bachelor's degree and a new, fulfilling job.

Are you socially embarrassed with people you're not familiar with? Be yourself, there's only one of you on this planet. Professionally, evaluate both your short-term and long-term goals in life. In general, feel good in your own skin. Popeye said it best, "I yam who I yam." If not, our sense of perception and reality fades and our computer fails us. Our perception can be grossly distorted and exaggerated by becoming anxious, fearful, confused, angry, or feeling pain and unhappiness in our lives. The brain needs reassurance, someone to bounce our thoughts off of. That's why we seek out family or friends to talk things out. That's one reason coffee breaks, happy hour, and cocktail parties are so popular. I've often said that the majority of the patients I've seen over the years are seeking reassurance, whether mental or physical. Doc, does mom have Alzheimer's? No she's alert and passes the mini mental exam. Doc, my face is drooping on one side, am I having a stroke? No, it's Bells Palsy (swelling of a facial nerve) and with treatment it will heal nicely.

"THE THREE LITTLE PIGS"

APPLYING COMMON SENSE TO OUR FRAME (MUSCULAR-SKELETON SYSTEM)

Perhaps the 'three little pigs' can help us out on understanding our frame. The only pig to survive in the framing business was the one who made his house out of bricks. Though we are all born with a basic brick frame (muscular-skeleton), it's how we go about maintaining and conditioning it that matters most. It all begins with the type of fuel (food) we use to nourish it. Calcium and protein rich foods (dairy and vegetables) are necessary to ensure a healthy framework. Unlike a rigid brick structure, our frame is mobile and flexible. As with all mechanical frames with moving parts, our joints require a delicate touch of lubricant (synovial fluid) and routine range of motion. Some of our joints are extremely complex, like our shoulder joint, which rotates in three different ranges (rotates, extends vertically and horizontally). Others like the sacral-iliac joint (located in your pelvis) have limited movement. Some functions of our structure (bones) include the manufacturing of our red blood cells and immune system. With all those functions, common sense requires us not only watch what we eat, but properly engage in a daily routine of stretching your muscles, ligaments and tendons.

To energize the majority of your frame, simply incorporate a lot of daily walking, cycling, or other fun physical activity (running, swimming, tennis, golf or dancing to name a few) into your daily routine. It's nonsensical to spend your extra time lounging on a couch. Inactivity works against every aspect of your muscular-skeleton system. It was designed to move with activity, and any disuse leads to atrophy and weakness of your muscles, ligaments, tendons and osteoporosis (thinning of the bones). Use it or lose it. Many of my geriatric patients, with a history of inactivity, have taken up pool therapy, or are inspired to take daily mall walks.

Why does our muscular-skeleton system fail us at times? Lets go back to the pig's brick house and imagine adding ten additional floors to the house. Guess what happens to the base floor? It begins to weaken with all that additional weight, causing the mortar to crumble, bricks to compress, break down, and eventually the pig is left with an unsafe house—not any better off than his unsuccessful brothers. That's exactly what happens to our frame when we become obese, especially the damage it does to our hips and knee joints. Even as an observer you'll notice how an obese person's gait wobbles from side to side and their lower leg deviates to a lateral position. This type of gait translates into an erosion of the cushion (meniscus) in the knee joint and deterioration of the hip joint. Obesity needs to be addressed early in life. Like the sign in the china store states, "you break it, you own it." The tragedy I've witness over the years is seeing young obese patients coming back as adults' years later, requiring knee and hip replacements. It's an accident waiting to happen. Lifestyle changes are in order *now*, not later.

Over usage (aggressive repetitions) of your joints should be minimized as much as possible when swelling and pain persist, though your work environment may demand it if you are to keep your job. This is especially true with loaders, bricklayers, drywall workers, and heavy construction workers. Many employers will reassign workers to a different job description if possible, or retrain them in a job that doesn't involve physical stress. Accidents involving injury to the bones (fracture) or joints (ligament and tendon tears) need immediate care (think of RICE—rest, ice, compression and elevate) along with treatment by a physician.

Finally, over time, all mechanical devices wear out and may require new parts. As with an old car, its not going to last if you keep racing and abusing it. Some parts of our frame may become diseased (arthritis) or weaken with thinning of the bones (osteoporosis). Others parts like our muscles disappear (sarcopenia), some of which is due to inactivity, but primarily due to age. Remember, the three mechanical medical problems we all face in life evolve around our frame—back and neck pain, arthritis, and difficulty walking. Common sense then tells us though we can't turn back the clock, we can continue with a proper diet (calcium and protein rich), maintaining daily physical activity, keeping in touch with our physicians with regards to our medications and possible need for joint replacements, and avoiding any repetitious activity that is painful.

"HEARTBREAK HOTEL"

A COMMON SENSE APPROACH TO OUR BODY'S PUMP (HEART) AND PIPES (VESSELS)

Unlike a strictly mechanical device, like a water pump, our heart has an emotional side to it…thus the term "heartbreak," as in Elvis's "Heartbreak Hotel" song of "since my baby left me." It responds to our fears and the general stresses of our daily lives. These responders come in the form of hormones (adrenalin-fight or flight) and nerves (vagus—from the brain). Somewhat akin to a pump receiving unregulated surges of electricity, the heart may beat irregular and/or rapid. Cardiologist, Dr. Robert Elliot found heart muscle in fit young fighter pilots literally shredded in uncontrolled fatal crashes from the extreme stress of facing certain death. I recall a similar incident with a couple that had been married for over 50 years. The husband called to say his wife had just died and requested an ambulance. When they arrived at their house, they discovered he too had died of a heart attack.

Just like the pipes in our homes, our vessels (pipes) can erode, leak and become plugged (atherosclerosis), similar to pipes in our homes that become overloaded with sludge. Autopsies on young army soldiers fighting in the Korean War revealed advanced hardening of their arteries (atherosclerosis), in part due to their diet (fatty

36

foods of the 50's), their DNA (component of our chromosomes that carries our genetic information), and the stress of the battlefield.

Back in the 60s, I had a 26-year-old die of a heart attack with no previous symptoms. He had an average cholesterol level, but unfortunately was a heavy smoker and overweight. He died on a Saturday, his busiest day as a barber. His parents had no known heart problems, but lived a relatively stress-free life on a small farm. The smoking, drinking, poor eating habits and stress was more than his heart could tolerate.

What then is the common sense approach to keeping our heart and vessels healthy? To begin with, not all hearts and vessels are created equal. Much depends on your DNA, which we have no control over. Like being dealt a lousy poker hand (a pair of threes), some of us have a family history of early heart attracts and require an aggressive medical workup. Similar to maintaining a water pump, your heart also needs constant care. That means starting good eating habits in the pre-teens years, along with daily exercise, and the avoidance of smoking and drugs.

Though we are all generally aware that daily exercise, a healthy diet, and the avoidance of smoking and drugs are beneficial to maintaining a healthy heart, we have a tendency to wait for a life threatening event to happen before doing what we already know is good for our heart. Besides, most of us are in constant denial about our health, thinking it's always someone else whose going to have the problems, not us. It's like the wildebeest grazing in the Serengeti assuming the stalking lion is focused on the furry guy next to him.

Therefore, common sense strongly suggests we keep our DNA history up to date, being aware of not only our parent's medical history, but also our grandparent's and their siblings. With one in three American adults having some form of cardiovascular disease, it becomes our most-feared health concerns. With the thought we might become the next victim of a heart attack, we can easily become paranoid. I received a phone call in the 60's at 2AM from a colleague complaining of chest pain, and asked if I would meet him at my office. In those days there was no 911 or ER services available in our area. After a thorough exam and EKG, all tests proved negative. His history showed he had just attended a weeklong medical conference on heart attacks. Once I assured him that his heart was okay, his chest pain immediately disappeared.

Aside from being aware of a family history of heart disease, daily exercising, maintaining proper eating habits and avoiding poor habits like smoking, alcohol or drugs, you may ask, "What other common sense approaches can I take?" For starters, take an enteric-coated baby aspirin a day. Aspirin interrupts the platelets ability to form clots in your heart arteries. The exception is for those allergic to aspirin, asthmatics, and those with bleeding disorders.

Now for those who already have coronary artery disease or hypertension, there are effective treatments available. Bypass heart surgery (attaching a patient's healthy vessel to bypass the blocked heart artery) or implanting stints (small mechanical tube) into the coronary arteries has been successful, but for the majority of patients with hypertension and heart disease, the pharmaceuticals are preferred. Aside from aspirin, which aids in avoiding blood clots, there's statin drugs (Lipitor, Crestor) that have been proven to lower cholesterol and slow down plaque buildup in the heart vessels. The majority of hypertensive treatments include beta-blockers (Bystolic, Tenormin), to calm down the heart rate, ace inhibiters (Altase, Prinivil, Catpopril) that decrease hormone (Vasopressin) activity in the kidneys and diuretics, which in turn reduces excessive fluids in the body.

"GOING GREEN"

COMMON SENSE FUEL AND AIR FOR OUR DIGESTIVE AND RESPIRATORY SYSTEM

In this world of going green, we are constantly looking for the most efficient usage of our engines. It saves us fuel and money. Yet as humans, we are extremely inefficient at fueling (food) our bodies. We not only use contaminated fuel (trans fats, saturated fats, and sugar), we end up flooding our engine (body) with too much fuel (food). This not only shortens the life expectancy of our engine (body), but also causes it to run rough (lack of energy, fatigue, and shortness of breath). In their desperate quest to shed weight, obese patients frequently seek out the latest fad, diet or pill. My response would be "perhaps a one-way flight to Ethiopia would be a better choice."

For an engine to run, it requires fuel (gas) and air (oxygen), but not too much of either and not contaminated. Likewise, our bodies too require fuel (food, which is processed in our digestive system), and air (oxygen that is extracted by our lungs). There is probably more print devoted to the variety of fuel (food) for our bodies than any other subject matter on this planet. It runs the gamut from the best place to get it, how much it costs, who prepares it best, which is best for your health, how frequently do you need it, and when to use it. The list goes on and on.

With that said, how then do we best incorporate the common sense factor into our digestive and pulmonary systems? Perhaps, it's by keeping the analogy of "going green"—using food more efficiently and maximizing our body's life expectancy. There are several choices before us. The thousands of diets and gimmicks we're exposed to daily can influence us, or we can take a common sense approach. Lets begin with our digestive system. Historically, over the last tens-of-thousands of years, our diet has been wild grains and wild meat. However, since the industrial revolution, we've processed our food to appease our palates—namely adding an abundance of sugar, fat and salt to our food. I would frequently tell my patients you could add salt and sugar to garbage and it would be edible. I recall many of my younger patients asking me why they get so wired when drinking up to a dozen sodas or energy drinks a day, and is it a problem? My response was, "Come back in a couple thousand years and perhaps by then our bodies might have adapted to such extreme abuse." I'm not suggesting we go back to our caves and eat wild fruits and grains, nor am I suggesting we never indulge in an occasional treat. Life needs relaxation and fun too. If your engine specifies high octane gas but none is available and you put in a lower octane, I'll assure you it will still run, but not as well. Common sense requires some degree of discipline, so don't be temped to always use the cheap gas for your engine or only the junk food to fuel your body on a regular basis.

So then, what's a practical and sustainable fuel for our bodies? Start your day with what I call a dog food approach…namely eating the same food daily for breakfast. It can vary slightly, however, an unadulterated grain cereal (shredded wheat or rice) with skim milk (or soy) sprinkled with your favorite fruit (banana or berries) is a good start. If your dog could talk, he would tell you that with all that natural fiber, his bowels are regular, and his body weight remains steady. I also suggest adding a diluted (half water, half juice) glass of grape juice (vitamin C and antioxidants) with your breakfast. Avoid making your meals complicated or rigid. For your next two meals of the day, lean towards vegetables, fish, white meat and fruit. Avoid fried foods and fats. Allow yourself some fun food once or twice a week, otherwise you might become frustrated and fall back into old eating habits. Fortunately today, many fast food establishments offer options other than burgers and fries, such as salads, and fresh sandwiches. It's a big help to avoid calling all this a diet. We break diets over a period of time, simply put; they are all doomed to failure. Over the past four plus decades, I've heard every diet out there—south beach, east beach, north beach, and west beach to the son-of-a-beach. Let's just rephrase it as a "healthy routine" we bring into our lives, or better yet, a "lifestyle change".

As with the air filter on your car, which keeps dust and dirt from interfering with the efficiency of your engine, your respiratory system requires the same respect. A better diet does little if you contaminate the air (oxygen) going into your lungs with smoking. You can't have it both ways and expect your engine to perform at maximum efficiency. If you feel doomed to failure on any of these issues, then I suggest you spend five minutes in front of a mirror and have a serious conversation with yourself, and decide if you want the glass of life half empty or half full. If you compromise your health and continue to smoke, then you have to live with a half empty glass. Don't look for gimmicks or sympathy to weasel your way out of turning your life around. The time is now, not tomorrow, or next year. I recall a young female smoker who attempted to stop smoking on several occasions, only to fall back to her habit again. On follow-up visits, she would apologize to me for her failure. I had to correct her; it was *her* lungs that were being damaged, not mine! She finally got the message, and stopped. Sadly, on another occasion, a middle-aged man with a long history of smoking two packs a day came to see me with a recent history of weight loss over the last four months, which is suspicious for cancer. After completing a full history and physical I took a chest x-ray, and found a large tumor in his lungs. After explaining the findings, I referred him to an oncologist (Dr. specializing in cancer treatment). When he left the office, he tossed his cigarettes into the trash can. Unfortunately for this smoker, it was too late. He died six weeks later.

"THE BIRDS AND THE BEES"

TOO MUCH NONSENSE ABOUT
PRODUCTION / REPRODUCTION
(SEX)

In our everyday lives, we're exposed to the miracles of both reproduction (sex) and production (growth/building) of both the living and the things we make. Just watch the TV program "How's its Made", and you witness our ingenuity in reproducing the same item identical to the original production model, be it a car or a toothbrush. Even more complex is what we witness in nature, both in the plant and animal kingdoms. Whether it's a small redwood seed growing into a gigantic tree, or the small fertile egg growing in a human mother, common sense has little to do with it.

There is common sense, however, when we apply reproduction (sex) to our lives. Our sex drive is second only to our drive to eat. Like eating, it's pleasurable; otherwise we would never continue our species. With our larger brain, we are the only living animal that have reproduction forefront in our minds 24/7, with perhaps the exception of pigeons (joke). This is especially evident with the proliferation of sexual images in the media, be it movies, TV, magazines, books, or the Internet. Unfortunately, when that exposure overrides common sense, our lives can be forever changed—unwanted pregnancies, sexually transmitted diseases, addictions, depression, anger, rejection, low self-esteem, broken relationships, etc. You can avoid many of these negative outcomes by recognizing your own personal weaknesses, and seeking professional counseling to help you avoid unwanted exposure to manipulated ideas of sex, such as pornography. It's a bit like placing a diabetic in a candy store, and telling them not be to tempted to stray from their diet.

Over the decades of practicing medicine, I've found infidelity to be the single biggest cause of broken marriages and relationships. Many of the macho TV beer commercials frequently emulate the coolness of drinking and picking up on whoever is available. Even with the best attempts of sex-ed in our schools, sexual relationships amongst adolescents is over 50% in some school districts. It becomes a right of passage for these kids. However, sex involves more than teaching anatomy and physiology, yet with that limited exposure, I've treated young girls who literally thought they could get pregnant by oral sex or kissing.

The phrase "too young for motherhood" is something we generally think of in third world countries, where young girls are forced into early marriage, or sold into prostitution rings. Making my daily rounds at our hospital one day, I was ambushed by the obstetrical nurse saying "Dr. Cosh, quick, come with me! I need your help! Someone has dropped off a young pregnant girl and left. She's fully dilated and we need you to deliver her." In the process of delivering the baby, I was attempting to extract as much history from her as possible, including her age. When she answered twelve, the nurse and I both were dumbfounded, only to be shocked further when she said this was her second baby. Children should not be mothers—period. The nurse and I witnessed first hand how these atrocities to children are not exclusively relegated to third world countries.

There's also a strong emotional aspect relating to sex, primarily with regards to females. I have counseled many young girls over the years, who were devastated by guilt and hurt over a sexual encounter, and left to deal with their emotional pain.

Maintaining a healthy sex life includes an open dialog with a partner, avoiding discussions of old relationships or failed sexual exploits, and most importantly, keeping a balance in your life—staying physically active, strengthening social relationships, staying focused on your career and keeping a sense of humor. Case in point: One evening, I was volunteering at a homeless clinic in downtown Denver, and a middle-aged male patient said he had an embarrassing personal problem. I reassured him that I'd seen and heard about everything, and that I'd be more than happy to help him. The next words from his mouth were "I have a tick on my dick." I had to suppress the smile on my face, only because he said it so poetically. I proceeded gingerly to remove one gorged tick. Thankfully, this was before Viagra.

"REMOVING RUST"

USING COMMON SENSE
WHEN FACING BODY RUST
(CANCER)

We are all aware of what rust can do to our bridges, vehicles and boats. In fact, its corrosive and deteriorating effect on steel is not too far removed from what cancer cells do to our bodies. One of the most difficult situations I've faced in my four decades of practicing medicine is telling patients they had the "C-word"—cancer. Patients in general will correlate cancer with painful long-term treatment and death. And yet, all cancers are not the same. The complexity of cancer is as variable as the stars in the sky. Some skin cancers are superficial, grow slowly, and are easily treated, with little threat to the patient. Melanomas are not in this category. I've personally lived with skin cancer for over forty-five years. I'm also a two-decade survivor of prostate cancer. Others are aggressive and dangerous, such as pancreatic and certain forms of brain cancer. However, in our modern world of technological advances in medicine, cancer treatment (oncology) is improving literally on a daily basis, and even with the most aggressive type of cancers, new treatments might be available for you. Today, it is more common to say you are *living* with cancer, instead of *dying* of cancer. Just like repairing your rusty car, the earlier one seeks repair (treatment) for the damage done, the better the chances are for a successful outcome.

A patient's common sense is to seek help from their physician as soon as their body tells them something is wrong. If you have unexplained weight loss, fatigue, lumps, sores, pain, or blood from any source other than cuts, it's a good idea to use that common sense and seek medical attention, as these can be signs of cancer. Beware of family or friends, though well meaning, who reassure you not to worry, and that everything will be fine. A middle aged female patient of mine, who was diagnosed with lung cancer, and under the care of an oncologist, was responding nicely to her treatment. A year into her treatment, I received a call from her stating she was short of breath, and had lost fifteen pounds. She said she quit her therapy for the last three months, because an aunt from another state told her she would be healed by prayer alone. Six weeks latter she died. Prayer, plus wise judgment with your medical care, is paramount in treating cancer.

When a physician approaches a patient with the C-word, they also need to use common sense. They must allocate enough time with the patient and their family to discuss their case, on a personal, face-to-face basis. The physician should never delegate this duty to a staff member. Until a definitive diagnoses is established, the physician should be extremely cautious in over utilizing the C-word with the patient. Otherwise, they're adding unnecessary stress to the patient and their family.

A patient's shock and denial are the two issues a physician deals with when explaining how cancer will affect their life. Compassion and empathy will lessen a patient's stress level, and allow the patient to listen to your treatment program and prognosis with an open mine. Without that approach, the patient may develop a brain freeze and only hear cancer=death.

Once a patient accepts the diagnoses, and feels like an active participant in the treatment program, the prognosis improves, and the patient's life can move forward.

Is There A Doctor In The House?

CHAPTER 4

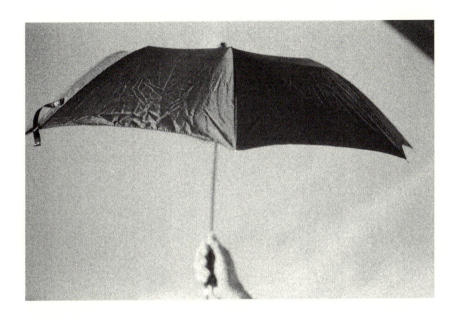

HOW EVENTS AFFECT OUR DECISIONS ABOUT OUR HEALTH

We're all aware how our plans can be affected by the weather. In many ways, our health, and life itself for that matter, are not much different than the weather—unpredictable and constantly changing. We become upset when bad weather interferes with our plans; somewhat like a bad cold or injury. This is especially true when the meteorologist promises sunshine and it rains instead, similar to when the physician tells us you can't play tennis this week because your knee isn't healed yet. When we're young, we feel invincible, even immortal. Then we're told we have a chronic disease, like diabetes, or worst yet, cancer. All of a sudden, we find ourselves in the middle of a fierce storm, like a tornado or a flood, fighting for our life, and we don't feel so invincible anymore. Our mortality stares us in the face. We need to be realistic about our future, and know that like the weather, storms do enter our lives at times, and we need to be prepared to handle those issues with sound judgment and action.

The very basic need to support our families and ourselves requires us to go to work. It becomes a major priority in our lives. Work pays for our food, a roof over our heads, and the ability to enhance our quality of life. Naturally, when health issues interfere with our ability to work, we often sacrifice our health in favor of work. We instinctively do this out of fear of losing income or our job. The downside of this reasoning is if you're infectious, you risk getting your co-workers sick too. The added stress weakens your immune system, and prolongs your recovery time. Recovering from surgery, fractures, cardiovascular events, or psychological problems take time to heal, and work often interferes with progress toward recovery.

Many years ago, I treated an elbow fracture on a patient who was a successful high school wrestler. He pleaded with me to allow him to wrestle the following day in a state match. It wasn't just any match. In fact, it would qualify him for a college scholarship. I had to explain to him that the broken bone had no idea what he was thinking, and that there would be future matches in his life. I assured him, risking permanent injury wasn't worth any scholarship. Sometimes the best workout can be *not* to workout. This isn't just true if you're sick.

 Even if you're fatigued, not sleeping well, or just generally run-down, bypassing a workout can be many times more beneficial than any workout would ever be.

For some activities, not going 100% can allow your participation without compromising your health. For example, if you're a singer in a choir and a bit under the weather, use your common sense, and don't sing at full voice.

Think of yourself as a pilot, and your body as your plane. Would you fly your plane into bad weather, unfamiliar territory, or with insufficient fuel or equipment? Of course not. Just the same, don't overextend your body and put it into harms way, and don't be afraid to ask for help. If your plane was running out of fuel, you'd radio the tower to find the nearest runway. If your body is running low on sleep, ask a friend to run that errand for you. This concept applies just as significantly to our health. Don't overextend your capabilities.

Is There A Doctor In The House?

CHAPTER 5

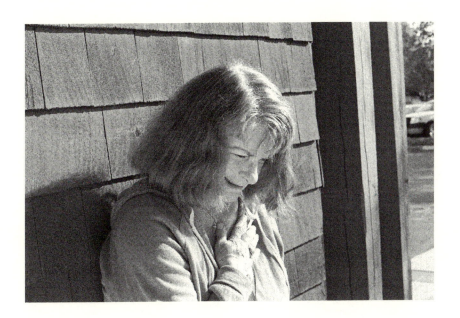

USING COMMON SENSE WHEN
DEALING WITH PAIN AND FEAR

Aside from the pain that brings a patient to my office, it is also the fear factor of what's causing the pain; is it a heart attack, stroke, cancer, infection, etc? The seven most frequent complaints I've treated over four decades of practice involved emotional, throat, chest, ear, back, stomach, or head pain. I will attempt to address each of these complaints with a little common sense, both with a preventive and treatment approach, in addition to a story or two, to make a point. Again, this isn't meant to be a paradigm for everyone, but a simple guideline to follow with your healthcare provider.

EMOTIONAL PAIN
A COMMON SENSE APPROACH

This is the granddaddy of all pain…bar none! It strikes at the very core of who we are. Only our individual tolerance can gauge to what degree we can handle the everyday crisis we are inevitably faced with. Much of our emotional pain is rooted in our genes, our environment, physical condition, and whom we associate with. Our status in life also influences us emotionally, and determines how secure we are in our own skin. This is true with both family and at the work place. The work place especially can push our buttons to our emotional limits. One of the most popular newspaper comic strips today is Scott Adams', "Dilbert," which illustrates this point best. From a recent strip, the pointed head boss walks into one of his employee's cubical, and says "I want you to work from home for two days per week to reduce our carbon footprint." The employee shouts "Noooo!" and says, "My wife and three children are in that house. They are mean to me." Whereupon the boss says, "How bad could that be?" The employee responds, " Let me put it this way. I'm sitting in an egg carton and talking to a moron, and is this better?" Most of us would rather absorb the pain and keep quiet if our boss gave us an order we didn't wish to carry out, though our thoughts would be more close to Scott Adams' cartoon character.

Emotional pain exhibits itself in many different forms: depression, anxiety, anger, irrational thinking, over generalizing, panic attacks, obsessive-compulsive impulses or recurring thoughts. These can possibly develop into a neurosis (a mental disorder involving distress), psychosis (loss of contact with reality), schizophrenia, or a borderline personality disorder, to name a few.

For the most part, we can all relate to periods of being down or fearful at times, but when it becomes a pattern and affects our ability to cope on a daily basis, we need help. Our demeanor changes, we find ourselves not using our seat belts, eating excessive amounts of junk food, or skipping meals. Why? Because the pain of depression is so great that you don't care about the consequences of your actions. We don't care if we get hurt or even die. During the early 60's, as an extern (medical student) making daily rounds at the hospital, I encountered a husband who was staying at his wife's bedside literally 24hours a day. She had a stroke. I assured him she was doing well and perhaps he should go home and get some rest. However, he insisted on staying at her bedside. On the forth day of his constant vigilance, he said, "I don't feel well," and collapsed. Despite extensive CPR (cardio-pulmonary resuscitation), he died. His depression was more than his heart could take.

You might feel that you're the only one experiencing these feelings, but you're not alone. Just walk in your neighborhood at night, passing house after house, and those people are most certainly experiencing similar interpersonal conflicts, some more extreme than your own.

Adolescents, are more susceptible to exaggerated degrees of mood swings because of their hormonal changes, incomplete brain development, and peer pressure. When these young patients would mention their wild mood swings, I would reassure them that it was similar to when their parents took them to the ocean as a child. They would hold your hand and walk you through the mild surf until you had the confidence to do it on your own. Later, when you entered adolescence, you took on the bigger waves, and got knocked around like never before—just like your daily moods. I'd assure them that once they got past the big waves, as an adult, things would eventually calm down. Although they would still occasionally be bounced around in life, they would eventually find balance and confidence in their lives.

So how does common sense enter the picture when it comes to dealing with the stress of emotional pain? As with all pain, we want it to stop. During medieval times they relied on leaches to *ease* their emotional pain and illnesses – thus the word dis·*ease*. Today we no longer use leaches, but instead *ease* our emotional pain by relaxing and engaging in fun activities.

When your emotional tank is running on fumes, it is not the time to take on the weight of others. A good start is to avoid being overwhelmed with the personal problems of friends and family, and to deal with your own emotional baggage.

When your emotional threshold becomes overbearing then you need to distract or redirect those feelings and negative thoughts. It's like changing the subject when you're arguing with someone; you divert the uncomfortable subject matter to a more pleasant one. To lessen your emotional pain, avoid the people, environments, jobs or fears that cause you pain. Reflect back when you experienced a painful emotion (being teased) in kindergarten. You can still recall it, but it's been diluted by time, and hopefully you've moved ahead with your life. A distraction can be drastic; you're angry with a co-worker and not sleeping well, but are informed you've won the office lottery pool. You're now less focused on the co-worker, and insomnia is no longer a problem.

Perhaps the best approach to treating emotional pain is engaging in daily physical activity. It has been proven to be effective with every type of stress disorder, including anxiety and depression, according to the American Psychological Association. Having written tens of thousands of prescriptions in my forty plus years of practicing family medicine, perhaps the most significant prescription I wrote was for bicycling, published in my book 'A New Customized Prescription For Cycling.' Whether it's a daily walk, jog or a ride on a bike, get active with a daily fun activity. The reason is it reduces stress. One of my patients was going through a stressful divorce, and discovered biking gave him the relief he needed. Recently, an NFL football player who was released from his team said, "I need to get away by myself, and ride my bicycle." It probably served him well.

As with any pain, if it doesn't go away, you need to be evaluated by your physician. Treatment for mental illness today offers a wide array of new and effective medications, coupled with support groups for all types of emotional problems. Frequently, patients placed on a psychotropic medication will say, "Doc, I'm not crazy, and I don't want to get hooked on any medicine." My explanation doesn't involve insanity, but how our newer medications are designed to assist the brain, when it's been either over or under stimulated. It doesn't imply that they will require it for an extended period of time, no more than staying on pain medication does when the pain is gone.

SORE THROAT
A COMMON SENSE APPROACH

We can all relate to experiencing an occasional sore throat. It's the nature of the sore throat that confuses us. Is it due to an infection (virus or bacterial), allergy (nasal, food or medication), weather (humidity), sinus drainage, spicy food, or perhaps straining your voice? Probably the cause that strikes the greatest fear in us is having strep throat. This type of sore throat is caused by a bacterium, known as group A-beta hemolytic streptococcus. It products a toxin that can play havoc to many parts of the body, including the heart (rheumatic heart disease). The general red flag that it might be strep is when there's a sudden onset of chills, fever (over 100 degrees), painful throat, tender swollen glands in the neck, and known exposure to a confirmed case of strep. Getting a throat culture, or rapid strep swab, is imperative. If a physician cannot see you right away, request a staff member or lab technician to perform one. After-hour options include going to an out patient facility. Some pharmacies and grocery store clinics are available to perform throat swabs, and treat if positive for strep.

One of my duties as chairmen of the hospital infectious committee was to perform routine throat cultures on all surgical personnel. Many who turned out to be strep carriers were completely asymptomatic. I recall a family that I frequently treated for strep. The only family member not seen was the mother, who stayed behind in the waiting room. She became a bit defensive when I asked to swab her throat, primarily because she denied having a sore throat. As it turned out, she indeed was the carrier. Pets too, can be strep carriers.

Waking up with a sore throat without a fever typically is caused by sleeping in a room with extremely low humidity. This is especially true in motels and hotels that are heated and cooled with systems that dehumidify the room air. Ideally, our sinuses function better when the humidity is between 40% and 60%. Travelers flying into either very high or low humidity environments are most at risk, like traveling from Florida to Arizona. The viscosity of our sinuses changes, allowing the lining of our throat to dry and be exposed to irritants, viruses and bacteria. If you live in a dry environment, purchasing a humidifier for your bedroom will help avoid those morning sore throats. If you are in a motel or hotel and that can't provide you with a humidifier, turn on a shower for 15 minutes prior to sleeping. Keeping a nasal bottle with saline solution in it will allow you to spray your nasal passages throughout the day when encountering extremely dry conditions, such as flying on airplanes.

Sore throats associated with allergies can be treated with cortisone nasal sprays that are dispensed by your physician.

Your physician must evaluate any sore throat that doesn't respond to simple gargling (with dilute salt water or lozenges), or is associated with neck swelling, difficulty swallowing or breathing, or lasts beyond several days.

EAR PAIN
A COMMON SENSE APPROACH

Nothing gets the attention of a parent faster than their child crying at 2 AM, because of an earache. Ear infections (otitis) are common in children, and need to be evaluated by a physician. However, you can offer some immediate relief by gently pressing the child's head against your shoulder, and applying a warm compress to the affected ear. In addition, an analgesic (Motrin/Advil) may be given. Ear drops, such as Auralgan, may also bring some relief and help calm the child down, until seen by your physician. Many a night, during the 60's, and prior to the availability of emergency room coverage, I would meet the parents and child at my office to treat the sick child.

A blocked ear canal cannot only be painful, but may also cause diminished hearing. A waxy substance called "cerumen" causes the blockage, commonly known as earwax. It's frequently caused by prolonged exposure to high frequency sounds. Unfortunately, the old axiom "don't put anything in your ear bigger than an elbow" isn't always followed when it comes to removing earwax. I've treated more than one ruptured eardrum, which was pierced by a bobby pin or toothpick. The simplest approach in removing earwax is with an over the counter irrigating bulb and wax softener such as Debrox. Keep the water in the bulb at 95-100 degrees F. If all else fails, your physician can syringe it out. Performing this procedure on a youngster on one occasion brought laughter to the family and myself.

While syringing the youngster's left ear, we noticed water coming out of his right ear! It wasn't from my forceful syringing, but residual water from his right ear.

Aside from removing earwax from the ear canal, I have also removed, paper, sand and insects—including a nest of spiders. Ear pain or hearing loss associated with trauma or a foreign body in the ear canal requires immediate evaluation by a physician.

CHEST PAIN AND CONGESTION
A COMMON SENSE APPROACH

The pain that gets everybody's attention is chest pain. It has an ominous association with an impending heart attack and possible death. As the leading cause of mortality, and morbidity, there's good reason to fear it. Why? Because it's indiscriminating; regardless of your gender, race, age, intelligence, wealth or religion, it can strike. To help differentiate the nature of the chest pain let's review the common forms of non-cardiac pain first. Remember, there are no absolutes with chest pain.

Generally, chest pain that can be reproduced by pressing on the chest wall or by a twisting rotation of the upper body is usually from the rib cage. This is especially true if you can recall stressing your upper body over the last several days. Your memory from a week ago may be fuzzy, and hard to correlate with your present pain. Case in point: a mechanic complained of tender chest wall pain on his left side, and denied any action he performed in the last week which could have caused the pain. After further questioning, he did recall leaning against the fender of a car for several hours, replacing a power steering unit. As it turned out, that was the origin of his pain.

This is also the case if you're recovering from a chest cold that was accompanied by strenuous coughing. We expect to cough when we have a common cold. Coughing is the body's way of clearing unwanted pathogens (virus and bacteria), pollens, and other foreign material from our throat, trachea and bronchus. Any OTC (over the counter) pain medication can ease this type of pain, along with applying warm moist packs (no heating pad) to the affected area. For the most part, we can correlate the cause and effect for the majority of our coughing episodes. For example, we would expect some coughing following exposure to dust or pollen. This is usually more prevalent in the spring. Experiencing sinus problems, or exposure to rapid changes in humidity, can also produce a cough. Generally, using a humidifier and taking a cough medication (dextromethorphan/guaifenesin) will take care of most coughs. Sipping on ice chips will also assist in suppressing these types of coughs. However, coughing that is accompanied with chills, fever, chest pain, and or difficulty with breathing, requires medical attention.

Another common type of non-cardiac chest pain we commonly experience is after eating a heavy, fatty meal, which will typically show up as pain under the chest wall. However, this pain doesn't always deter patients from eating fatty, gaseous foods. I had a policeman who refused to give up his sausage sandwiches, knowing full well he'd be moaning with gas, later on. This is a fullness or sharp type of pain, which can be helped with an antacid, like Alka-Seltzer.

However, any form of chest pain that goes unabated, needs to be evaluated immediately by a physician.

Chest pain that requires immediate attention is when it feels like a heavy, crushing pressure across the chest wall (like an elephant stepping on your chest). Any chest pain accompanied with extreme weakness, faintness, nausea, and/or sweating, requires an immediate 911 call and the taking of an aspirin to minimize clot formation.

Not all heart attacks involve chest pain. My wife and I were in the middle of the Pacific Ocean on our way to Hawaii to attend a medical meeting, when a flight attendant asked if there was a doctor on board. I followed him to the front row of the cabin, where a large, middle-aged man was slumped over in his seat, while his wife screamed that he'd just had a heart attack. I quickly cleared out four seats, and with the assistance of several passengers, laid the man down and proceeded with CPR. Slowly, I got a pulse and stabilized him for the remainder of the flight. I later received a nice letter from his wife; informing me her husband never experienced any pain, prior to slumping over. She thanked me and said her husband was recovering nicely.

STOMACH PAIN
A COMMON SENSE APPROACH

We frequently use the term "quit your bellyaching" when we are tired of someone constantly complaining. And yet, that's exactly what stress does to our belly—it causes it to ache. When we are relaxed eating a meal, our gastrointestinal autonomic nervous system is in what's known as "parasympathetic mode." This means our digestive juices are allowed to flow, and our bowels to move (peristalsis), thereby maximizing the bowel's ability to absorb nutrients into our bloodstream. Conversely, if we are upset (stressed) while eating, our mouth becomes dry; we chew less, eat faster, and are more likely to choose foods high in fats and sugar. We want comfort foods to help us overcome the stresses we're experiencing, because they make us feel better in the short term. Our gastrointestinal system is now in an "autonomic sympathetic mode." This is when our digestive juices cease, and the bowels slow down, creating spasms and gas buildup, all of which cause pain in the stomach. In the mid 50's, I had just departed Davis-Monthan Air Force Base in Tucson, Arizona, on a flight to Phoenix. After leveling off at 2400 feet, I was checking my map, when suddenly my peripheral vision caught something in my windshield. Quickly looking up, I saw a C47 (DC-3) making a climbing right turn right into my airplane. I immediately pushed the control stick forward and to the left. As my right wing rolled over, I could see the rivets on the fuselage, missing it by inches. After landing the plane in Phoenix, I went in for lunch at the airport restaurant. Needless to say, my turkey sandwich tasted like cardboard, and all the water in Phoenix couldn't wash it down. Why? My gastrointestinal system completely shut down, from my near death experience.

Even though we frequently say the brain constantly talks to our gastrointestinal system and our gastrointestinal system talks to our brain, the gastrointestinal system has it's own independent nervous system. It's complex, and little understood when it misfires. Everything from what enters it, our genetics, age, gender, immune system, overall health, stress level, and environment are factored in when evaluating it. I recall a middle aged woman years ago, who was convinced she had colon cancer, because of a strong family history of colon cancer. Although she didn't experience any symptoms of cancer, my gastroenterologist screened her, and found no evidence of cancer. She continued her annual colonoscopy for over a dozen years, with normal results. It was perfectly normal and correct for her to follow up with annual exams. However, her daily obsession with colon cancer distracted her from enjoying life. It was as if her brain and colon couldn't come to terms with each other.

Common sense would suggest not eating when you're upset in order to avoid a stomach ache. In truth, life doesn't always work out that smoothly. When things are out of control in our lives, we need some assistance. It may come in the form of common sense decisions, like avoiding noisy fast food establishments, allotting more time to eat, choosing a friend to share your meal with, or avoiding mixing work (texting and phone calls) with your meal.

Chronic digestive problems can be helped according to what part of the gastrointestinal system is involved. The beginning of the digestive system, including the mouth, can be helped with proper dental care and hygiene. The stomach and esophagus, where acid reflux occurs, can be treated with over the counter acid reducers (pepcid), or antacids (Maalox). Smoking, alcohol, spicy foods and soft drinks all aggravate acid reflux.

Problems in the lower gut, which includes the small and large intestine, is where we can experience either hyperparistalsis (cramping and diarrhea) or delayed peristalsis (cramping, gas and constipation). One condition we frequently hear about is IBS (irritable bowel syndrome). It's usually associated with older woman, where their bowels vacillate between constipation to diarrhea. Maintaining a high fiber diet, or taking a fiber supplement (Citrucel, Metamucil) on a daily basis, will remedy most of these problems. For short periods of time (less than a week), Pepto Bismol or Imodium can be used to control mild cases of diarrhea. This is assuming you're not running a fever, having blood in your stools, or not experiencing relief from your symptoms.

All other gastrointestinal concerns that don't resolve with conservative therapy require an evaluation by your physician.

BACK PAIN
A COMMON SENSE APPROACH

Our evolutionary progress hasn't quite caught up to our vertical stature. We are still in the process of becoming a permanent biped-or two-legged creature. Our back muscles, vertebrae, ligaments and tendons, have not yet developed the ability to withstand the daily rigors of walking, bending over, and lifting heavy objects. It's no wonder when we add emotional stress to the formula, we see a full 1/3 of the population with some form of back pain. I recall patients with a history of back pain experiencing spontaneous spasms in my office, while describing a stressful situation to me. They literally turn white with pain, because of the overwhelming stress in their lives.

Back pain roars it's ugly head in as many forms as we have parts of our backs. Back pain occurs when our vertebrae (the bones comprising our spinal column), compress our discs (the pillow-like cushions in between our vertebrae) against our spinal cord (nerve). This causes back pain that radiates into our legs (sciatica nerve), along with weakness and numbness in the affected leg. Injury is more apt to occur when you're obese and not physically fit. A majority of back injuries I've treated are the result of improper lifting techniques. Instead of lifting an object off the floor with their legs and keeping it close to their body, they're more apt to lift with their back. This increases the tension on the back muscles, ligaments (tissue holding our bones together), and tendons (tissue attaching our muscles to our bones), and rotates our back while lifting an object. It's somewhat akin to rotating the towers of a suspension bridge, and overstressing the cables, until they snap.

Common sense dictates a conservative approach initially. This includes avoiding strenuous activity and prolonged periods of sitting. It's a good idea to rest (semi-reclined, with legs flexed) as much as possible, apply cold packs (15 minutes three times a day) to the affected area for the first day, followed with warm moist packs (30 minutes-two times a day for up to two weeks), and no heating pads (dry heat increases inflammation). If possible, take OTC (over the counter) Advil/ Motrin/ Aleve (not only reduces the pain, but also reduces the inflammation) for pain, as needed. Muscle relaxants aren't that helpful because of the side effects (dizziness). Gentle back stretching and manipulation can also help as the pain lessens a bit. The above recommendations can also be applied to muscle and ligament tears or contusions.

Perhaps the most frustrating aspect of a back injury is the perception that it will be gone in a short period of time. Not so! We've just damaged a large part of tissue that supports our body. We're aware of how long it takes a sprained ankle to heal. Multiply that by a factor of five, and you realize your back is going to require additional time and patience to heal. Many patients want instant relief, and resort to gimmicks (vibrators, heat packs, stretching machines, magnets, etc.) for a quick cure. Beware of doctors promising relief with 10 trips to their offices, or surgeons who are quick to suggest surgery. They will not only drain your pocketbook, but also interfere with your ability to properly heal.

Some back injury patients with busy schedules want to negotiate a treatment plan, other than the ones just mentioned. Case in point: A 36-year-old man, with a family (wife and three children), was on vacation in another state and injured his back. His schedule called for him to drive his three children back home for school the following day. Because there was a 12-hour drive involved, I suggested his wife drive, while he reclined in the passenger seat, placing ice packs on his back (storing back-up ice packs in a cooler) on the trip home. In addition, I suggested taking Advil as needed for the pain. He agreed not to work the following week, and to follow up with his physician.

For the most part, those of us who have injured our backs will bite the bullet and cancel any previous commitments. On the night prior to flying to Chicago to attend a medical meeting I was scheduled to speak at, I pulled my back, resulting in much pain. It was only after confessing "Doctor, heal thyself", that I wisely cancelled the trip.

However, excessive pain (Greater than 5 on a scale of 10), prolonged pain beyond several weeks, weakness, or prolong numbness of the extremities, dictates an evaluation from a physician, and possibly more aggressive treatment options. Second opinions are advised when surgical intervention is being contemplated.

HEAD PAIN
A COMMON SENSE APPROACH

When we become angry with someone, we might tell them, "You're giving me a headache!" Headaches are so commonplace in our lives that we sometimes take them for granted. Physicians are so used to hearing the complaint, that the term "take two aspirins and call me in the morning" is used as an offhanded joke, but headaches are not a joke to the person having them. They can be so painful that some early tribes in Africa would have their medicine man (witch doctor) use a crude circular saw (trephine) to cut through the skull to allow the evil spirits to escape. Frankly, the two aspirins sound like a better option.

Fortunately, the majority of headaches are not life threatening, and can be alleviated with pain medication (aspirin, Advil or Aleve), massage, and cold packs to the back of the neck (10 minutes two times a day as tolerated), and staying in a darkened room. For the most part, these types of headaches are brought on when the neck and scalp muscles are under excessive tension, usually caused by stress—conscious and sub-conscious. Simply applying pressure to the temporal (side of the head at eye level) area or base of your skull will produce pain. A middle-aged female patient, with no previous history of headaches, came to my office complaining of morning headaches over the last two weeks, involving her temporal and neck area. She denied having any personal problems, but after further questioning, she said her mother-in-law from England was scheduled to visit for two months. We then spent some time discussing a plan that would address the issues she was worried about. She called back a week later, and the headaches were gone. This is a good example of a headache from sub-conscious stress.

We have four sets of facial sinuses, all basically surrounding our eye orbits. The largest are the maxillary, just under your cheeks. The frontal are located just over your eyes. These sinuses, in addition to the smaller sphenoid and ethmoid, serve to add mucus to your nasal passages, thus adding humidity and trapping dust, pollen, and germs from entering your lungs. When these passages from your sinuses to the nasal area become blocked, pressure builds up and you feel pain, usually around your eyes. When they become infectious, you may also run a fever, and should see your doctor. Aside from over the counter pain medications (Advil, decongestions, nasal spray moisturizers), applying warm moist packs over the effected areas, and inhaling moisture through the nose, will help alleviate the discomfort. Unfortunately, your genetics may have given you large sinuses, and you may be programmed for chronic sinus headaches. In that case, a rhinologist (specialist of the nose) can surgically alleviate headaches by opening the passages between the sinus and the nasal compartment.

Headaches associated with severe head trauma, especially those involving unconsciousness or memory loss, require immediate evaluation by a physician.

Certain types of headaches require your physician's attention. They include chronic headaches (more than two per week, and not responsive to over the counter pain medication), and headaches associated with visual changes (flashing lights or aura, temporary loss of vision and/or hearing and nausea). The latter may indicate a migraine headache. A sudden onset headache that is one-sided, usually around the eye, with tearing and redness, probably suggests a cluster headache. Scheduling an appointment with your physician is paramount in diagnosing and treating these types of headaches.

Is There A Doctor In The House?

CHAPTER 6

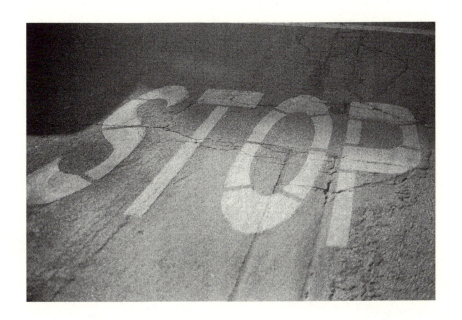

WHEN COMMON SENSE ISN'T ALWAYS
COMMON SENSE

The adverb "always" encompasses a vast amount of territory, and therefore must be clarified, especially when applied to one's definition of what common sense is. Everyone has a different understanding of common sense, and let's face it, not everybody has the aptitude for good common sense or when to use it. It's somewhat like fine wine—age adds to its value, but gulping it down can lead to disaster. Case in point: A pilot flying in turbulent weather at night becomes lost. Rather than relying on his navigational instruments, his common sense tells him to fly where he thinks the airport is. Instead of proceeding south, where his instruments tell him the airport is, he goes east, where his sense of direction tells him to go. He runs out of fuel and crashes.

The same thing occasionally happens in medicine. A patient complains of experiencing mid-back pain for several weeks. The physician diagnosed it as disc disease. A CAT scan (an imagining machine) confirms the diagnoses. Seems like a simple case of common sense diagnosing (mid-back pain=disc disease). However, the patient's back pain continues, despite treatment for his disc disease. The physician queries the patient a bit further, and finds a strong family history of heart disease, and that the back pain became worse, especially when walking up several flights of stairs. In fact, the patient also had angina (heart pain, due to lack of blood to the heart muscle), which was later confirmed by a coronary angiogram (dye injected into the arteries of the heart). So initial common sense may not necessarily be common sense at all—which in medicine is called chasing a red herring.

We frequently refer to common sense as thinking outside the box. However, it's not an excuse for not initially thinking inside the box. Like the lost pilot, the physician needed to stay within the box a bit longer before assuming his/her common sense diagnosis was the right one.

CHAPTER 7

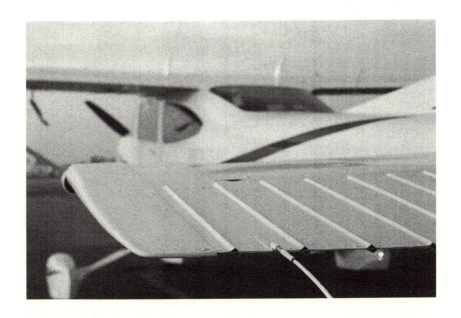

KEEPING OUR BODIES ON AUTO-PILOT

Having served as a Senior Aviation Medical Examiner for the FAA, I've had many airline pilots tell me that their autopilot does a better job flying and landing the airplane than they do. This is also true when it comes to how many of our bodily functions are regulated. Things like controlling our growth, our breathing, heart rate, the digestion of our food, and our metabolism are regulated without our direct control. This is accomplished in part by our hormones. Hormones are chemicals that act like messengers, sending signals throughout our bodies, regulating our metabolism (insulin, thyroid, growth hormone etc.), our sexual drive and reproductive systems (estrogen and testosterone), and our ability to fight or flee (adrenalin and catecholamine). They all have feedback mechanisms that interact with each other. Unlike other animals, humans can override many of these hormones. We can give growth hormones to youngsters that lack it. Insulin and thyroid are common hormones given to diabetics and hypothyroid patients, and list goes on. However, they can be harmful when dispensed improperly, especially to athletes who use them for performance enhancement.

To help fine tune these functions, we need to understand how our circadian rhythm (biological cycles) interacts with the overall health of our bodies. Every bodily organ has its own individual cycle for maximum performance. This is predicated on numerous physiological factors: optimum nutrition, adequate rest, maximum blood flow, and their ability to interact with each other. However this isn't always the case. Internal chaos occurs when different organs are out of sync with each other, like the liver and the brain. As a result, the patient feels fatigue, insomnia, irritability, or mentally foggy. People who work night shifts for extended periods of time throw off their circadian rhythm, because every organ hasn't adjusted to the lack of a full eight hours of sleep that they should normally get. This also occurs when we travel through several time zones. Say you fly from NYC to LA. When you arrive in LA, your mind sees it's only 6PM, but your body knows it's 9PM. You're out of sync. If your brain has been deprived of sleep, and the ability to dream, you become less focused, and more apt to make mistakes. A patient of mine recalled the time he was the copilot on a cargo plane landing in a South American city late at night. He said that both he and the pilot hadn't had a full night's sleep in three days. He wasn't aware of it, but the pilot fell asleep just before touchdown, resulting in a crash landing. Fortunately there were no fatalities. Sleep deprivation throws the whole circadian rhythm out of balance, and can result in dangerous outcomes if not addressed properly

Dreaming literally clears out the cobwebs, or cognitive underbrush, from your brain. Your brain randomly discharges during sleep, somewhat akin to the random firing of Chinese fireworks. That's what makes them so confusing to understand. Just don't overanalyze them. Though nightmares are unpleasant, they occur less frequently as we age.

For a basketball team to win, it needs all 5 players to be in sync with each other. The same applies to our bodies; when our liver, kidneys, heart, brain, and lungs are working at 100%, we feel sharp and on top of our game. Experiencing insomnia, eating poorly, being out of shape, or not taking your medication may cause your liver to dysfunction, which in turn alters your circadian rhythm, resulting in feeling sub-par.

Is There A Doctor In The House?

CHAPTER 8

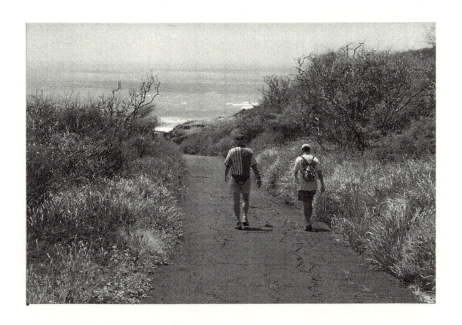

A WALK DOWN MEMORY LANE

Over the course of four and a half decades of practicing family medicine, I have many memories of unique situations I've encountered, ranging from the humorous to the serious. I trust by sharing a few of these anecdotal experiences, patients will better appreciate what their personal physicians have to deal with.

MY BAPTISM BY FIRE

I entered family medicine as a solo physician during the mid-1960s in a semi-rural area west of Denver. I thought I was prepared for anything that came through my doors. To keep my office overhead down, I hired a middle-aged woman, whose previous job was working as an office clerk. She had no medical background. I figured I could teach her all the medical nuances she needed for my practice, and besides, the minimum wage at the time was just $1.50 an hour! What I didn't anticipate was what happened on the second day of starting my practice.

It was extremely stormy, with winds gusting to 70 miles an hour. I was in the middle of examining an elderly man with prostate disease, when I heard screaming people running down the office hallway. While I had my gloved finger up this gentlemen's butt checking his prostate, the door flew open. There stood a man holding a blood-soaked, unconscious teenager in his arms. The old man getting his exam shot off my finger like a missile, quickly pulled up his pants, and left the room. I immediately had the man carrying the boy lay him on my treatment table. Apparently, the high winds had broken several large glass windows from their frames, splattering the broken pieces into the teenager. He had sustained lacerations from his head to his feet, and was in shock from the blood loss. After quickly starting IV (intravenous) fluids and oxygen, I asked the man to assist in applying compression to the lacerations. My untrained assistant I'd just hired helped me while I sutured the lacerations. Within a few minutes, I realized she was leaning on me, and then falling along the wall, painting a beautiful red line from her lipstick along the fresh white paint, before finally landing on the floor. Now I had two to care for, when the prostate patient popped his head up from behind a gathering crowd to ask when I was going to finish with him.

The good news is everybody survived, including my quasi nurse.

DEATHBED CONFESSIONS

The tragedy of hearing deathbed confessions is wondering why their issues weren't addressed earlier, when you could have possibly assisted them. I'm certain fear and embarrassment were the reasons why they weren't, for most of the cases. Like most physicians, I've heard more than my share over the years. I'll only address a couple. The first one that comes to mind was from a WWII veteran. He had terminal cancer, and said he wanted to get something off his chest before dying. He was a sergeant on the front lines in Germany near the end of the war. His encampment was guarded by a sentry, who was ordered not to allow civilians into the camp. Apparently, an elderly German woman and her daughter would pass the sentry post to get water on a daily bases, against orders to stop. Because the private at the post didn't enforce the order, the General ordered my patient, "Sergeant, I want you to replace that chicken private, and if that old German lady refuses to stop on your orders, I want you to shoot her!" The next day, the lady again refused to stop, whereupon he pulled out his 45 and shot her in the head. Visions of her lying in a pool of blood with her daughter crying over her never left him. Tears streamed down his face as he finally got the story off his chest.

The second confession was from an elderly lady with terminal heart disease. When she was an eight year old, she pleaded with her best friend's mother to allow her daughter to have a sleepover at her house that night. Reluctantly, she finally consented to allow her daughter to go. The next morning, while her friend was walking back to her house, a truck killed her. At the funeral, her friend's mother told her she was responsible for her daughter's death. She said she's carried that guilt her whole life, never having shared that story with anyone.

Hopefully, the non-judgmental comfort I gave to my patients eased their conscious a bit.

SOME DAYS ARE TOUGHER THAN OTHERS

Not all experiences in family practice are happy ones. This one occurred during my third year of practice. I was interrupted while seeing a patient by the screams of a new mother running into my office holding her dead baby. I quickly initiated resuscitation, and after what seemed like a half hour, there was no response from the child. Sadly, it was a crib death (SIDS...Sudden Infant Death Syndrome). I called the young father and had him come to the office. Both were devout Catholics, and asked me to call their priest to minister the last rites. Unfortunately, the priest said he was busy and couldn't come, and instructed me to give them. This was not my expertise, especially as a non-Catholic. I mustered up enough courage, and entered the treatment room with the grieving parents and prayed to God I could give them some comfort. Hopefully I did.

"WHAT'S ALL THE COMMOTION ABOUT?"

As a young doctor in the 60's, I'd delivered babies in motels (unplanned), twins in the back seat of a taxi stuck in traffic, and in a house as a volunteer in rural southern Colorado. I thought I had all the bases covered when it came to obstetrics. That was until the day I heard screams coming from my waiting room. It was from a young pregnant girl in labor, who wasn't a patient of mine. In the 60's we did not have 911, EMTs, or any other medical backup when emergencies occurred. As the only medical facility in my area, it wasn't uncommon for medical emergencies to end up in my office. After a brief history, she said she was only seven months pregnant when she went into labor. A pelvic examination revealed she was fully dilated, and the baby was presenting as a transverse lie (with one arm and leg in the birth canal), which is abnormal and makes for a difficult delivery. After a challenging delivery, I had to explain to a full waiting room what all the commotion was about.

PERCEPTION AND REALITY

Events in life aren't always what they appear, and that applies to medicine as well—perhaps even more so. While seeing a patient one day, I was interrupted by my nurse who said I had an emergency coming to the office. According to the mother, her youngest had just severed his finger off. When he arrived, I quickly examined his finger, only to find a small scratch and some dried blood. I assured the mother that his finger was okay, and went back to seeing patients. Later that same day, my nurse said that a plumber was coming in with a cut finger. On his arrival, I stuck my head in the room to ask him how serious it was. He said it was nothing to worry about, and that he could wait while I finished with my current patient. When I finally got to the plumber, I was shocked to see a completely severed finger! This was just after he'd told me it was no big deal…wow! Perception and reality: all in the eyes of the beholder.

LIFE IS NEVER FAIR

It's not every day I get to see a paradox between two similar patients. On one particular morning, I had the privilege of treating a young man with an ear infection. What made him special was that he was in a wheelchair and was blind. He was very friendly and appreciative of my treatment. Later that afternoon, I had another young man with a minor medical problem to care for. He too was in a wheelchair, but with perfect eyesight. However, he was angry and hostile, and said nobody was as bad off as him. I told him I wish he could have met my other young patient earlier. Perhaps using his eyesight, he could help that young man get about, and in return, that blind man could allow him to see how much he had to be grateful for.

STAYING UNDER THE RADAR

On the 13th of April 1987, I was assigned to cover the Colorado Capital as doctor of the day by the

Colorado Academy of Family Physicians. It was a volunteer program to assist members of the House that became ill. Unbeknownst to me, it was the same day Colorado Senator Gary Hart was scheduled to announce his quest for the Presidency of United States. The announcement was to be on the steps of the state capital. All the major news networks covered the event. I was assigned, with my black medical bag, to sit by the Senator. During his announcement, I said a small prayer that some crazy nut wouldn't show up and try to harm the Senator. The last thing I wanted that day was to be on national news treating an injured victim.

CONTROLLING ANGER AND REVENGE

When dealing with any type of personal conflict, one of the most difficult is revenge—to punish somebody in retaliation for harm done. One evening, I was alone in my office finishing up with paperwork, when one of my male patients walked into my office with a gun. He said he had just found out his wife was seeing another man, and he was about to kill both of them. After an hour of counseling with this distraught man, he agreed to get help, and then confessed he wasn't really planning to kill anybody, but just needed to talk to someone. Against my advice, after only a month of therapy, he said he and his wife didn't need any further help. I cautioned him that I sensed some residual anger, and said it would be a good idea to stay in therapy. I guess it didn't surprise me when several years later his wife came in my office sobbing. She had just received an out of state call from him saying he was shacked up in a motel with another woman, and now they were even.

Unfortunately, his simmering anger wasn't fully resolved, and his revenge did not make things even.

AN UNSIGNED DEATH CERTIFICATE

Shakespeare said, "We all owe God a death." With regards to the terminally ill, physicians often are pressured by family members to pursue untested treatment plans, or to overextend hospital stays, all in a bid to extend life at any cost. However, the opposite can also occur. During the 60's, I was covering for an on-call group, and received a call from a nursing home asking that I stop by and sign a death certificate on one of their patients. I asked the nurse what the time of death was, only to be told that the patient wasn't quite dead yet! I made a quick trip to the nursing home, and found a middle-aged female patient with a rapid pulse, a temperature of 105, and diminished breath sounds in both lungs. I had the patient admitted to the hospital with pneumonia, and discharged her to another nursing home several weeks later. The first nursing home was closed down after I reported this to the state health department.

CHAPTER 9

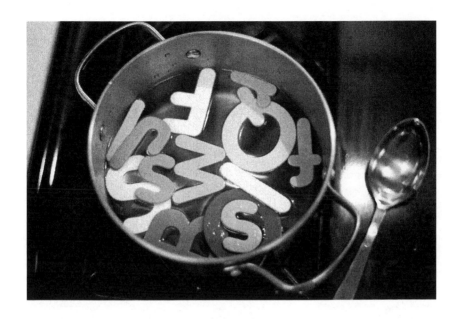

Although, we naturally assume it's the physician who does all the questioning, it's more often the patient doing the quizzing. I've listed twenty-six of the most frequently asked questions I've encountered, reflected by a word that best sums up a particular theme. Perhaps the best way of discussing them is over a bowl of homemade alphabet soup.

ALPHABET SOUP MEDICINE

A—Afraid

Patient:	*Doc, I'm so fearful*
Physician:	Normal, but we'll help you.

When a patient enters a physician's office with a new problem, they might perceive it to be serious and life threatening. One of the privileges of being a physician is seeing the relief on their faces when they've been reassured that it's an easily treatable problem.

B—Believe

Patient: *Doc, will I get better?*
Physician: Yes, with faith in your treatment.

With proper treatment, patients do get better, whether it's hypertension or diabetes. However, treatment of terminal cancer still requires faith in your doctors, and especially being open to possible new treatments. I had a middle-aged man diagnosed with a terminal brain tumor who was told he had six months to live. Three months into his treatment, he was offered to take part in a new experimental treatment program. Two years later he was still able to enjoy his family.

C—Commitment

Patient: *Doc, it's too hard to do*
Physician: It's a must to succeed.

Whether being treated for an infection or heart disease there are some inconveniences to deal with. A young diabetic years ago couldn't commit to taking his insulin and maintaining his diabetic diet. Over the years he lost his legs and vision and eventually died years later.

D—Denial

Patient: *Doc, I don't think it's serious*
Physician: We need more information.

It's only natural to question any news that threatens our lifestyle; whether being discharged from a job or told you have to have surgery. Early in my practice I saw a new patient with a large melanoma on his back and informed him it required immediate attention. He said he would look into it after his vacation in another month. Unfortunately, it was his last vacation.

E—Empathy

Patient: *Doc, are you sympathetic for me?*
Physician: To be objective, I'm empathic.

To make clear and accurate medical decisions physicians need to separate their personal emotions from what's best for their patients. Somewhat like a pilot with a cabin full of passengers, his first obligation is flying the airplane.

.

F—Failure

Patient: *Doc, I never fail to listen to you*
Physician: I promise not to fail you.

One of the pleasures of practicing medicine is witnessing the positive change you've made in a patient's health, whether it involved them giving up smoking or complying with their diabetic program.

G—Good

Patient: *Doc, I feel good now*

Physician: That's good to hear.

Giving immediate relief to someone in acute distress is usually followed by "Doc, I feel good now." I've heard this from many patients, ranging from a young boy after removing a foreign body from his nose, to an elderly female patient after lancing a large abscess.

H—Health
Patient: *Doc, I want to stay healthy*
Physician: I'll keep you informed.

Staying ahead of any potential medical problem is the key to good health. I've often said preventive care is worth ten times more then the treatment for the problem.

I—Inconvenient
Patient: *Doc, I don't have time for this*
Physician: It's not an option for you.

Somehow the word inconvenient has a ring of arrogance about it. It's not inconvenient to pick up your paycheck, but it is when dealing with your health issues. A mother once cancelled her sick daughter's appointment because she found it inconvenient to cancel her hair appointment.

J—Joy
Patient: *Doc, I'm missing happiness*
Physician: You need a balance in your life.

Happiness can't be bought. It comes from within. Adding some diversification to your daily routine, will allow you to see life from a different perspective. A middle-aged executive told me he needed a change from his daily routine and was basically unhappy. Upon asking him what made him happy, he said as a teenager he enjoyed washing his car. I said perhaps this is a good day to clean your car.

K—Kindness

Patient:	*Doc, you've been thoughtful*
Physician:	I appreciate your kind remarks.

A touch of compassion and kindness transcends barriers. The kindness I received from treating the medically underserved was more than I could have ever imagined.

L—Laugh

Patient:	*Doc, I don't laugh anymore*
Physician:	Let's help your depression.

Chronic depression is one of the most challenging medical problems physicians are faced with. Without fun and happiness in one's life, there is no laughter. Aside from counseling and medication, I would frequently suggest watching a silly movie, like one from "The Three Stooges."

M—Moderate

Patient:	*Doc, how do I find balance?*
Physician:	Cutting back is a good start.

More isn't always better. When you cram a 28-hour day into a 24-hour day something has to give. It usually equates to more stress in your life. A middle-aged female patient was seen over the Christmas holidays with a chronic back strain. She was holding down three part-time jobs, caring for her four children and volunteering at her church. After carving out a new schedule for her, the back problem was gone.

N-Normal

Patient: *Doc, am I normal?*
Physician: Normal has a wide range.

It may be normal for a cave explorer to squeeze between rocks, but extremely abnormal for a claustrophobic. Generally, people go out of their way to blend in with the crowd. If their friends are wearing a pink hat, they too will wear a pink hat. If their friends have a tattoo, they may also have one. You will be normal when you're at peace with yourself.

O—Outlook

Patient: *Doc, can you predict my outcome?*
Physician: Every case is different.

We all heal at different rates. With an elderly diabetic, it may require two weeks for an abrasion to heal, while with a healthy youngster, only three to five days. Generally, following the treatment plan with a positive attitude, will help the outcome to be successful.

P—Patience

Patient: *Doc, I have none.*

Physician: It takes time and patience.

True patience is judged over the long term basis, not short. We've accepted that there are sixty seconds to a minute. NASA engineers are patient when they are counting down the final ten seconds before launch, otherwise hitting the launch button three seconds prematurely would destroy the rocket. When patients prematurely stop their prescriptions, they are putting their health at risk. They need patience to complete the course of treatment.

Q—Quandary
Patient: *Doc, I'm confused.*
Physician: It's okay to be puzzled.

Life itself is complicated without the physician further confusing the patient with medical terminality their not familiar with. During my internship, the cardiologist I was assigned to was attempting to explain to the patient in technical medical language that he had suffered a heart attack. After what seem like an eternity, he asked the patient if he had any questions. The patient said, "Hey doc, did I have a heart attack?"

R—Resolute
Patient: *Doc, how do I remain steadfast?*
Physician: With personal determination.

It's difficult enough when you have a bad day when you're feeling good; imagine what a bad day feels like when you're going through chemotherapy or recovering from surgery. That's when you have to dig deep into your reserves and go with the flow, rather than becoming angry and resentful. Remember-this too will pass!

S—See

Patient:	*Doc, see I told you so.*
Physician:	I'll be more attentive.

As physicians, we too are subject to oversights. This is especially true when a patient tells you that the previous medication you had given them years ago didn't work, and then we have the audacity to ask them to try it again.

T—Tenacity

Patient:	*Doc, how will we succeed?*
Physician:	Be persistent and stay the course.

The game isn't over until you cross the finish line. Some treatments simply take longer than others. Treating hypothyroid disease may take three months or more before the patient notices any improvement. After casting a teenager's arm for a wrist fracture, I told her to make another appointment in two weeks and to call if she had any problems. She missed the appointment, and rescheduled a week later, only to also miss that one. I called her and she informed me that the wrist felt fine, and had her friends cut the cast off. Needless to say, she broke it again two weeks later. Stay the course.

U—Upset

Patient:	*Doc, this news disturbs me.*
Physician:	I understand, we have a plan.

It's human nature to become upset with unpleasant news, especially when it affects your health and future. As with all sad news, there are options for addressing the problem. Once you pass the shock stage, there's the acceptance phase, where you commit to a treatment plan that will allow you to heal and move forward with your life.

V—Viewpoint

Patient:	*Doc, do we need help on this?*
Physician:	We will seek other opinions.

With the rapid advances in medicine it's virtually impossible for physicians to stay abreast of every new treatment plan that is available. Family physicians are constantly conferring with their specialist on a regular basis. It's paramount, if we are to give optimal care for our patients.

W—Weary

Patient:	*Doc, I'm so worn out.*
Physician:	Understandable.

Not only our bodies wear out, but also our emotional state can reach a point of collapse. That's why you constantly require proper eating habits, a life balanced with fun and relaxation, exercise, and enough sleep. Don't allow your gas tank to go to empty.

X—Xeno

Patient:	*Doc, I never heard of this before*
Physician:	I'll research it.

The physician doing my college physical abruptly excused himself from the treatment room during the exam. He returned with a smile on his face several minutes later, explaining he had to look up a word on the physical that he wasn't familiar with. There's no excuse or shame in admitting you need help in finding the answer for something you're not knowledgeable or familiar with.

Y—You

Patient: *Doc, I worry about everybody*
Physician: Let's focus on your problems.

You, the patient, already have a lot more on your plate than you can handle, and yet you're constantly taking on everybody else's problems. Obviously, that's an unfair statement. Why? Because it's natural to be sympathetic to your family and friends. However, you can serve them better when your plate is in check. Get your own house in order first.

Z—Zest

Patient: *Doc, I can't get out of this rut I'm in*
Physician: Add some joy to your life.

Years ago when the phonographic needle was stuck on a defective record you would have to physically lift the needle off the record and reposition it. The same applies to the rut your in, reposition yourself out of it, buy a bike, take a walk, shop, go to a museum, fly a kite, get a pet, call an old friend, see a movie, enjoy a snack, etc…

CHAPTER 10

COMMON SENSE SUGGESTIONS FOR A MORE
BALANCED AND HEALTHY LIFE

Sometimes we're so consumed with the basics of
surviving in our day-to-day world, we tend to lose focus
on the direction our lives are taking. Periodically, it's
helpful to take time out for a course correction, and
update our agenda. Though there's a multiplicity of
other factors to consider, I've found the following
common sense suggestions can lend assistance to our
physical, mental, emotional and spiritual lives. We are
more than the sum of our parts. By challenging
ourselves in these areas, we can reevaluate our lives,

and make corrections that will give us that inner peace we all strive for.

I've treated many successful and wealthy patients, who were, by all external appearances, happy. In actuality, many were miserable inside. To achieve their personal goals of success, they shortchanged their families, friends, and ultimately, themselves.

MAKE FAMILY A PRIORITY

The word "family" can include many people— parents, children, relatives, friends, co-workers, teams, organizations and military units, especially those with shared combat experiences. Family brings security to our lives, hence the term "family support"—someone to watch our backs. As we've all experienced, it's when times or events are not so good that we see who we can call family.

Over the years, I've heard many tragic stories of families overcoming personal strife and staying together. One involved an elderly Polish man who not only lost his wife to cancer, but also his business in the same month. He told me how the family support he was receiving reminded him of when they endured the winter of 1939, when they were escaping the Germans. He recalled how each family member put their shoulders into the spokes of their wagon wheels, pushing them forward in the frozen mud. That was his definition of family. Family is a unit of people able to share emotions, feelings and memories. This is especially true during anniversaries and holidays. When you hear Bing Crosby sing "I'll Be Home for Christmas," the first thing most people think of is their family. With good parenting, a child instinctively will mimic the values their family has and blossom. If a caterpillar is denied foliage, it fails to become a beautiful butterfly.

Family can also have a dark and sinister side to it. People often fill the void of not belonging to a family by joining a gang. Members consider themselves family, but with far different ramifications—loneliness, depression, fear, suspicions and distrust. A young girl told me how her 18-year-old brother died at the hands of another gang. She said he enjoyed the prestige of the gang over his family. He traded the love of his family for what he thought was respect from his peers.

For the majority of us, it's the combination of all our families—our parents, children, grandchildren, friends, and our faith, that can make life so fulfilling.

HAVE A MORAL COMPASS

Morality, as we define it, relates to one's character, and the ability to make the distinction between right and wrong in life. Genetics and DNA are not factors in choosing your values in life as much as the environment you grow up in. Morality, or the ideas of what's right or wrong, are generally learned from an individual's family, schools, religious teachings and friends. In the absence of those influences, the line between right and wrong often gets blurred. A gang member would see nothing wrong with robbing someone, while most people would never think of such an act. The "Golden Rule" of treating others as you want to be treated is not just defined by your words, but by your actions. Morality has been diluted in some cases in order to serve the interests of the individual, and not your fellow human being. This blur is justified by some, who see an act of dishonesty or cruelty as right, because they had been mistreated themselves. A married policeman would frequently boast about all his sexual encounters while under my care. When I asked him how it affected his marriage, his response was his first wife betrayed him, so that his present infidelity was justified. I explained that his justification was based not on morality, but on his flawed reasoning that one negative action justified another negative action.

Human history has a long line of atrocities committed by those whose moral road was paved with a twisted view of right and wrong, resulting in untold devastation and death. A truly moral person feels a sense of peace when taking the high road in life, because it inevitably benefits his fellow man, rather than causing harm. That in turn results in a happier individual. We should all be cognizant that our God and society rewards those taking the righteous path. It allows for a restful night's sleep.

VALUE YOUR HEALTH

Ideally, we all wish for our bodies to be free of disease and pain. Unfortunately, as we age, time can become our enemy. To a child time moves slowly, somewhat like driving at 10 MPH. Later, as an aging adult, it quickly accelerates to freeway speeds. Usually, it's our face that reflects our age; however, realistically we need to acknowledge all of our organs are aging. A diseased liver (cirrhosis) is deceived by the youthful face of an alcoholic. Along with infections, accidents, and our DNA, poor habits play a major role in our health. Middle age is when we begin to get a wakeup call as disease begins to show it's ugly face. Years of bad habits, like smoking, overeating, lack of exercise, drinking, and drugs makes the body susceptible to a number of diseases, including those affecting the heart, liver, lung, and neurological systems. While attending a state medical meeting years ago, I witnessed one of our distinguished members being honored for his many years of service. After physically struggling to the podium, he gasped, "If I knew I was gong to live this long, I would have taken better care of myself." Don't let his words fall on deaf ears; implement your life changes now.

Environment also plays a role in acquiring disease. Factors like sun exposure (skin cancer), extreme temperature exposure (frostbite and heat stroke), pollens (allergies), insects and animals (infections and attacks), and the landscape (drowning and accidents) can all have adverse effect on your health. Gradually over time, our bodies begin to shut down. It's a natural process that affects all living things. The effectiveness of our organ systems slowly diminishes until death. The late cardiologist, runner, and author, Dr. George Sheehan (*Running and Being)*, said to maintain your physical conditioning as you age, would eventually require more time working out than there are hours in the day. Obviously, that's not possible, but it *is* possible to maintain some daily activity. Remember, age doesn't wear you down, disease and disuse do.

We are most vulnerable to infection in our early childhood and in our senior years. As we progress through life, each age bracket has it's own risk factors—accidents and childhood diseases in the young and cardiovascular disease and cancer for the elderly. Though we can't control our DNA, we can affect our chronological age (someone's real age) by staying physically active, eating healthy food, and lowering our stress levels. Our physical age will then exceed our chronological age. The best example of this I can recall involved a mother and daughter. They wanted to be seen in the examination room together. The younger looking one was sitting on my treatment table when I entered the room, while the clearly older looking one was sitting in the chair. I immediately embarrassed myself by addressing the patient on the table as "the daughter." Quickly looking at both charts, I was dumbfounded to find that it was the mother on the treatment table, not the daughter! The mother was 92 years old, while the daughter's age was 71. An extensive history from both patients revealed the daughter had been a two-pack-a day lifetime smoker and heavy drinker, with little physical activity, while the mother lived an active, smoke-free life on the farm. Although they shared similar DNA, the healthy lifestyle of the mother had her physical age less than her daughter's chronological age. The earlier we implement a healthy *lifestyle*, the further we extend our *lifespan*. This will only happen if the individual has the tenacity to stay the course.

HAVE A HOBBY

Hobbies are generally things we do in our free time. They allow us to forget about our day-to-day problems, and bring us joy. Many hobbies don't require a partner, or even physical activity. It may involve solving a crossword puzzle, playing solitaire, or restoring an old car. They provide a distraction that can reduce our stress levels, which can be as beneficial as exercise. Entertaining activities like going to the movies, plays, sporting events, amusement parks, or gambling casinos are but a few activities that help distract our minds from negative thoughts. These activities allow our brains a time out, so to speak—a chance to recharge.

Hobbies can also increase social interaction, which allows us an opportunity to talk out our daily frustrations or joys with others. After losing her husband, one of my patients began to withdraw from all social contacts and became depressed. She said her only joy was working with puzzles. I told her she might want to join a club at the local community center. She told me on a later visit that she had joined a group and had gained new friends. Her depression subsided. As with sports, it's important that hobbies not be taken too seriously, or they go from being fun, to a source of stress, thus defeating their initial purpose.

It is essential that we set aside sufficient time for activities. Don't feel guilty, or be made to feel guilty by others, because you took an hour out of your day to pursue your hobby. Just remind yourself that all work and no play can lead to an unbalanced life.

DEVELOP GOOD HABITS

Habits are repetitive actions we incorporate into our daily lives. Good habits sustain us, through good times and bad. Bad habits are usually the result of poor decisions and choices, many from a lack of mentors in our lives. Most of us know the difference between the good and bad. The habits we acquire in life begin forming during our early years, influenced for the most part by our parents, and to a lesser degree, by our peers. Over time, personal experiences help us form habits that hopefully assist us in making proper decisions. Habits affect what we eat, if we exercise or not, and if we have healthy sleeping patterns. Maintaining good habits requires a daily dose of discipline. We are often tempted to stray, either because of time constrains, or emotional stress. Stress is generally the catalyst that tempts us to stray into bad habits. This can translate into over-eating, drinking too much, smoking, or abstaining from physical activities. If the pattern continues, then we've gone from maintaining good habits to developing bad ones. However, we need to cut ourselves some slack when we occasionally slip up while trying to maintain good habits, and not lose sight of our long-term goals. Even as physicians, we can be hypocrites when we tell our patients "do as I say, not as I do." Many years ago, on a hot summer evening, I took my family to Baskin-Robbins for ice cream. While ordering an ice-cream cone for myself, I felt a tap on my shoulder. It was a patient, who said "Hey doc, you told me not to eat that stuff." Fortunately, my patient had a sense of humor, and acknowledged we had both slipped a bit. Another humorous example of physician hypocrisy occurred in the middle 80's at the Denver Children's Museum. Serving as the moderator (as President of the Colorado Academy of Family Physicians), along with a dozen family physician residents, it was our intention to give advice on proper eating habits to the hundreds of children and their parents attending the event. However, shortly after telling the audience to eat apples instead of junk food, I found the residents in the back room treating themselves to brownies.

Good habits lead one into the virtues of a fulfilling life. President Harry Truman had a healthy attitude for speaking the truth, even if it meant losing public support, as when he fired General Douglas MacArthur. History proved him right. He also maintained a daily habit of taking walks, and enjoyed a long, happy life.

Teenagers are especially susceptible to bad habits, partially because their brains aren't yet fully developed. Peer pressure may lead them into drugs or engaging in unprotected sex. It may be more difficult for them to be excluded from their peers than to resist temptation.

KEEP THE FAITH

Although religion implies an organized system of beliefs centered on a supernatural being, it's usually the individual's faith that defines their conviction and loyalty, more so than the religious organization itself. Without faith, religion is not much different than a social club, with a set of privileges and rules. Religions per se require their followers to abide by a code of conduct and rules. This is fine, as it provides a framework for believers to operate in, but it is faith that sustains a conviction without logical proof, rather than a set of rules. Alexander the Great had once said what he hadn't conquered or seen, didn't exist. Not much faith there. Today, when we enter into a building or fly on a plane, we have faith the engineers knew what they were doing, and we don't question their decision making. When we're alone or in danger, we gain comfort in placing faith in our God. That's because at some point in time we've experienced a similar situation where God's hand has helped us through a crisis. Faith then becomes your beacon of light.

I can say unequivocally, during my four decades of practicing medicine, that patients who exhibited faith when facing a health crisis appeared to have a higher rate of successful outcomes, and endured less stress during that time period than those who didn't. Years ago, I admitted an elderly patient with a massive heart attack to the cardiac unit at my hospital. She remained in critical condition for several days, with little hope of surviving. However, against all odds, her family and priest were vigilant with their daily prayers at her bedside. Just when there appeared to be no hope left, she slowly improved and lived for another decade. Both the family and the patient credited their faith to her recovery.

One testimony in particular caught my attention in the national news following the volcanic explosion of Mount Saint Helens in 1980. It was from a camper that survived the initial blast, and after nearly a week of being lost and without food, he felt he was going to die. Desperate, he prayed to God that if he saw a cross on the barren landscape, it would give him a sign of hope. Shortly thereafter, he spotted a lone tree with two branches that formed a cross. Within minutes, a helicopter appeared over the ridge and picked him up. Though the naysayers will explain it as a coincidence, they would have a difficult time convincing that camper otherwise.

CHOOSE A HAPPY VOCATION

Though it's true that many insects, like ants and bees, are programmed with different functions within their colonies, those functions are controlled by their genes rather than by choice. For example, there are ants and bees that guard the colony, workers that seek out food, and others, like the queen, that produce the young.

On the other hand, humans are the only animals that have the ability to generally choose what vocation they wish to pursue in life. For many, that choice has been denied, either by family tradition (business), gender (woman's place as the housewife), race (discrimination), or economics (unaffordable education). Fortunately, that paradigm is slowly changing, and vocational choices are becoming available to all, regardless of gender, race, religion or financial status.

It's been estimated that the majority of the workforce is unhappy with their job. For some, it's not so much the job, but the conditions and people they work with that causes this unhappiness. The fortunate minority is able to look forward to going to work daily. I recall one of my airline captains telling me how much he enjoyed his job and looked forward to the challenges it presented. Like marriage, or any other lifetime commitment, don't rush the decision to choose what you are going to do the rest of your life. Make it *your* decision, and not one that's meant to please someone else.

An executive from a large corporation came to see me after being laid off. He was devastated, and had no idea what he was going to do next. After asking him what made him happy, his response was "Painting." Years later he had a successful house painting company.

WORK TOWARDS A POSITIVE LEGACY

Our legacy is essentially the trail of dust we leave behind after we die—the good, the bad, and the ugly. Some leave a legacy of humility and compassion, like Mother Teresa, Sister Rita, and my late father, Clarion Cosh. I was blessed to have worked with Sister Rita, as my nurse, at the Samaritan House in downtown Denver for over a dozen years. Her 75 years of service to the homeless is an accomplishment few can ever match. My father was a coach and teacher at Vineland High School in New Jersey for over 35 years. He instilled values of compassion, discipline, faith, and service to community into his students. His legacy lives on because he lived the ideals he bestowed on others. Some leave a legacy of leadership and service to country, like Abraham Lincoln, Winston Churchill and Dwight Eisenhower. Of course, there are those whose legacy is one of destruction and fear, like Adolph Hitler, or Joseph Stalin.

Though we all stumble occasionally, making wise choices, based on our morals and values, goes a long way in securing a good legacy. Hopefully, your legacy will extend beyond your family, by touching the lives of your co-workers and friends. We can only hope our legacy of doing good trumps the bad in our life, and that the baton of good is passed on to make life more fulfilling for those who follow us.

CHAPTER 11

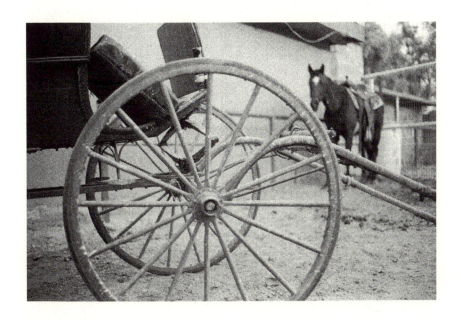

CIRCLE YOUR WAGONS

A generation ago, it was not uncommon to watch western movies with the likes of John Wayne leading the wagon trains across our western frontier. As nightfall approached, he would have them circle their wagons to create a barrier offering protection from any possible hostilities that lurked in the dark. With regard to protecting our health, our bodies also have built in barriers. The bodies' largest organ, the skin, does exactly that. It's a natural protective barrier against bacteria, viruses, and other pathogens from invading our bodies. Conversely, our individual body cells, the smallest unit of life, have a membrane that protects the cell mechanically and chemically from its environment. Human health is based on the function of maintaining our physical, mental, emotional, and spiritual well-being. Together, they coalesce into an inseparable unit. We can diagram it similar to "Leonardo da Vinci's Flower of Life's" geometric circles, each overlapping the other. Our four strongest barriers (wagons) protecting our health (flower of life) include a daily routine of exercise, proper eating habits (following the Department of Agriculture dish icon), fun/relaxation, and a restful night's sleep. Protecting your health starts now, not tomorrow or the next day. Forget the gimmicks and mirrors. Stay focused on the "Circle Your Wagons" icon—exercise, fun, eating habits and sleep. This requires a personal commitment to change your ways, or as Henry David Thoreau said "Things do not change; we change."

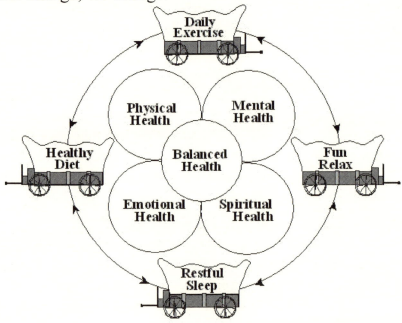

ABOUT THE AUTHOR:

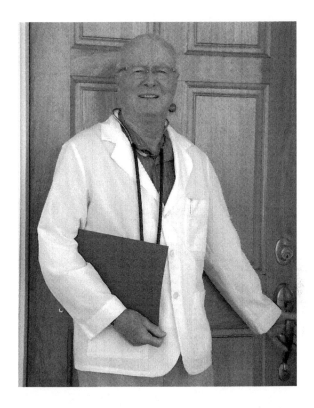

Dr. Cosh is a board-certified family physician, a Fellow in the American Academy of Family Physicians, a Senior Aviation Medical Examiner (Ret.), and Past President of the Colorado Academy of Family Physicians, with over four decades of family practice experience. In addition to his busy private practice, Dr. Cosh served the poor and medically indigent. Through his efforts, medical clinics were established at the Samaritan House, Jefferson Action Center, Manna Ministries, and Doctors Care. He is the founder of ClinicNet. He was recognized as one of the Super Hero's of Colorado Family Medicine, recipient of the 2005 Harold E. Williamson Award, the 2009 Alumni Service Award from Kansas City University of Medicine & Biosciences, and recognized by the Colorado State Senate in 2006. As an advocate of daily exercise, he has authored two books on cycling.

90329916R00068

Made in the USA
Middletown, DE
22 September 2018